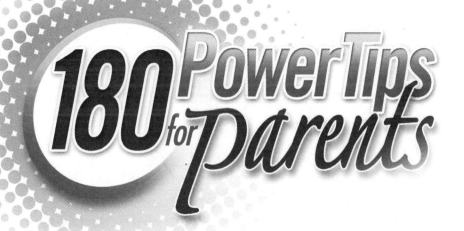

DR. KAY KUZMA

Other books by Dr. Kay Kuzma

- *Belonging: Overcoming Rejection and Discovering the Freedom of Acceptance* (Nancy and Ron Rockey with Kay Kuzma)

- *Between Hell and High Water—God Was There: Survival Stories From Hurricane Katrina* (Kay Kuzma and Brenda Walsh)

- *Easy Obedience: Teaching Children Self-discipline With Love*

- *The First 7 Years: Parenting With Strong Values and a Gentle Touch*

- *Mending Broken People: 3ABN Miracle Stories*

- *Parenting Boot Camp: Basic Training for Raising Responsible Kids*

- *Passionate Prayer Promises: More Than 100 Prayers and Scriptures That You Can Pray, Claim, and Believe* (Brenda Walsh and Kay Kuzma)

- *Prayer Promises for Kids: More Than 100 Prayer Promises to Pray, Claim, and Believe* (Kay Kuzma and Brenda Walsh)

- *Serious About Love: Straight Talk to Single Adults*

For information on Dr. Kay Kuzma's other resources, visit **www.FamilyResourceRoom.com.**

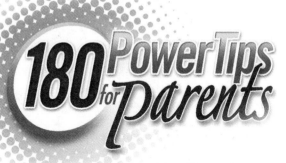

DR. KAY KUZMA

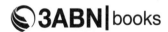

Pacific Press® Publishing Association
Nampa, Idaho
Oshawa, Ontario, Canada
www.pacificpress.com

Cover and Inside design by Chrystique Neibauer | cqgraphicdesign.com

The author assumes full responsibility for the accuracy of all facts and quotations cited in this book.

Additional copies of this book are available from two locations:
Adventist Book Centers®: Call toll-free 1-800-765-6955 or visit http://www.adventistbookcenter.com.
3ABN: Call 1-800-752-3226 or visit http://www.store.3abn.org.

3ABN BOOKS is dedicated to bringing you the best in published materials consistent with the mission of Three Angels Broadcasting Network. Our goal is to uplift Jesus Christ through books, audio, and video materials by our family of 3ABN presenters. Our in-depth Bible study guides, devotionals, biographies, and lifestyle materials promote whole person health and the mending of broken people. For more information, call 618-627-4651 or visit 3ABN's Web site: www.3ABN.org.

Library of Congress Cataloging-in-Publication Data

Kuzma, Kay.
180 power tips for parents / Kay Kuzma.
    p. cm.
ISBN 13: 978-0-8163-2499-6 (pbk.)
ISBN 10: 0-8163-2499-9 (pbk.)
1. Parenting—Religious aspects. 2. Families—Religious aspects. 3. Parenting. 4. Families. I. Title. II. Title: One hundred eighty power tips for families.
BL625.8.K89 2011
646.7—dc23

                                                                                            2011039916

11 12 13 14 15 • 5 4 3 2 1

How to Get the Most Out of Your Power Tips

Parenting is a twenty-four-hour-a-day job. Every minute is crammed with things that must be done for your family. But you can give only so much without refilling yourself with thoughts to help you refocus your priorities and reflect on what God may be trying to say to you through His Word.

That's why I've written this practical daily inspirational guide filled with power tips that can be read in less than a minute. Each practical suggestion is tied to a Bible verse that can change your life, if you will reflect on it and allow God's Spirit to impress you with how you can apply it. Remember,

Through wisdom a house is built,
And by understanding it is established;
By knowledge the rooms are filled
With all precious and pleasant riches
(Proverbs 24:3, 4, NKJV).

May this be your experience as you daily apply the wisdom, understanding, and knowledge of God to your family. One minute a day can change your life—if it's a God-inspired minute!

What Is a Family?

What does the word *family* mean to you?

Here's how some third-graders defined family. Janet said, "A family means a free apple, and you don't have to pay a five hundred dollar fine for a mistake." Sheila wrote, "A family is a place where you can play the piano without being shy." Corrine said, "When you have a family, you don't need anyone else but God."

What does your family mean to you? If your family means more to you than you've let them know in the past, maybe it's time to make sure that your love message gets through. Perhaps you'll identify with Louise Fletcher's famous lines:

> *I wish that there were some wonderful place called the Land of Beginning Again,*
> *Where all our mistakes, and all our heartaches and all of our poor selfish grief*
> *Could be dropped like a shabby old coat at the door, and never be put on again.*

Why not resolve today to start living each day the dream you have for your family? Dreams can come true.

Behold, children are a heritage from the LORD, the fruit of the womb is a reward. —Psalm 127:3, NKJV

New Week's Resolutions

When you make New Year's resolutions, do they last about a week, and then you're back to your old habits? The reasons may be that the resolutions are too general or too idealistic or that you make too many. For example, you decide you want to spend more time with the kids, lose weight, be on time to appointments, and never discipline in anger. There is no way anyone is going to keep all those resolutions!

The answer is to make New Week's resolutions, not New Year's resolutions. And make them specific. Say, "I will spend fifteen minutes each day with each child," or "If I am angry, I will go into my bedroom and pray before disciplining."

At the end of the week, you will have no doubt whether or not you have kept your resolutions. If you have, celebrate. Success for one week will spur you on to continue the next. If not, you may want to modify your resolutions and make them more realistic.

Why not make some specific New Week's resolutions today and see if it doesn't help change those bad habits into better ones?

I can do all things through Christ who strengthens me. —Philippians 4:13, NKJV

DR. KAY KUZMA

Making Family Appointments

If business appointments keep you from spending time with your family, perhaps you should start making appointments with your family!

Consider the example of Connie Giles, a busy executive. When her children wanted to do something with her, she would usually look in her schedule book and say, "I'm sorry, kids. I already have an important appointment."

One day her son asked, "Mommy, do you think I'm an important appointment? Why don't you write my name down in your appointment book?"

From then on she reserved time with her kids and wouldn't miss those important appointments.

Her children are grown now, but the times Connie remembers and cherishes the most were not committee meetings and conferences. They were the appointments with her children to go backpacking, deep-sea fishing, and star gazing.

Why not try what Connie did? Take out your calendar or schedule book and make the most important appointments of all.

To everything there is a season, a time for every purpose under heaven. —Ecclesiastes 3:1, NKJV

Team Spirit

How is your team spirit? I'm not talking about a football or baseball team, but your family. Does your family feel like a team? Or is everyone doing his or her own thing?

Deanne and her two kids didn't feel like a team. As a single mom, Deanne was overburdened with work, graduate school, and family responsibilities. Training for an up-coming marathon was what kept her invigorated. But her kids hated jogging, so they spent most of their after-school time with friends.

If Deanne didn't do something quickly to revive her team's spirit, they were all going to feel like losers. The answer was buying Rollerblades for the kids. Now they could look forward to spending time together with Mom while she was running.

If your family's team spirit needs bolstering, start doing things together! Start living for each other, not just for yourself. And make your home the most attractive and fun place on earth for your children. Team spirit gives energy, enthusiasm, and creative solutions to family challenges so everyone can be winners. It's essential in order to survive in this fast-paced world.

Make me truly happy by agreeing wholeheartedly with each other, loving one another, and working together with one mind and purpose. —Philippians 2:2, NLT

DR. KAY KUZMA

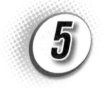

Who in Your World Needs a Hug?

It was only a sixty-second TV spot, but it scored. The scene: a typical American family rushing to prepare breakfast.

The phone rings. Sis grabs the receiver and dashes across the kitchen as she talks. Junior piles the toast high and heads for the table. *Crash!* He stumbles over the phone cord. Mom appears just in time to see the toast flying in all directions. She delivers an ultimatum, "The next one to spill anything is going to get a smack!"

Waving her arms for emphasis, she bangs into the glass of milk held by little brother. Milk splashes all over the floor.

Dad comes forward to administer the punishment. "Well, honey, it looks like you deserve a smack." He grabs his wife, raises his hand, and hugs her, then gives her a kiss with such a loud smack that the kids clap their hands and cheer.

The next time things get a little hectic and you're tempted to deliver an ultimatum, why not deliver a hug and a kiss instead and see what a difference it makes.

"Do for others what you want them to do for you." —Matthew 7:12, TLB

The Love Cup

We're all like love cups. When we're empty, we have nothing to share. But when we're full and overflowing with love, we have enough to give away—and we can be loving to others.

The hard part, especially for a child, is to keep the love cup full and overflowing in a world where cup emptying is so common. Criticism, rejection, looks of disappointment, being too busy, or harsh, angry words can quickly empty a love cup!

And because children equate love with attention, when they feel their love cups are empty, they often end up misbehaving in order to get a parent's attention. Care for them with kindness, show respect, accept them unconditionally, let them know they are forgiven, and trust them appropriately.

The cup-filling way is to give your family what they need. Give them some positive attention—a little love.

Fill them up until they overflow. And chances are that obnoxious attention-getting behavior will melt away, and they'll have enough love to give a little back to you.

"This is My commandment, that you love one another as I have loved you." —John 15:12, NKJV

DR. KAY KUZMA

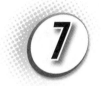

Making the Terrible Terrific

Every morning, rain or shine, Mom would greet her son with, "Wake up, it's going to be a terrific day," and together they'd go milk the cows.

One cold, windy morning, Jim rebelled. He said, "It's going to be a terrible day."

"Well," Mom replied, "if you think it's going to be a terrible day, you'd better stay in bed."

Sighing in relief, Jim dozed until he smelled breakfast, then dressed and went downstairs. "What are you doing?" Mom asked.

"I came for breakfast," Jim said.

"You can't eat breakfast. That would make it a terrific day." And she sent him back to bed.

He tried to come down for lunch but was again sent back. By dinnertime, Jim admitted that this was the worst day of his life.

"Well," said his mother, "it's up to you to choose whether you have a terrific or a terrible day. But you've got to work to make a day terrific."

I think that's great advice. Why not put a little extra into today—and make it a terrific one for your family?

And now, dear [parents], one final thing. Fix your thoughts on what is true, and honorable, and right, and pure, and lovely, and admirable. Think about things that are excellent and worthy of praise. —Philippians 4:8, NLT

Investing in Smiles

Usually when you give something away, it's gone. But it's just the opposite with a smile. Give it away and it multiplies.

One day Tammy's daughter complained, "Mommy, why don't you smile like you used to?"

At that moment there wasn't too much in Tammy's life worth smiling about. Then she remembered a home-finance principle she had learned: "Start saving when you have the least, and you'll be investing in the future." What if she started smiling when she least felt like it? Would her smiles multiply like money?

It didn't take her long to find out. Her daughter seemed happier, her office became a more cheery place, and her own life didn't seem so dreary.

A smile can't solve serious problems. Nor should it be used to mask troublesome emotions that need to be dealt with. But it's an investment that will multiple and offer some great returns. So, why not give it a try?

A glad heart makes a happy face. —Proverbs 15:13, NLT

DR. KAY KUZMA

Elevating Your Home Career

Kate Hanson used to be embarrassed when people asked her what she did. She didn't like saying she was "just a housewife," so she began to call herself a "family management and relational specialist."

Then when people would ask, "And what do you do?" she would explain that her job was to prioritize goals and work out a plan of operation so objectives could be achieved, thus fulfilling the needs of family members. "My biggest challenge," she would continue, "is with conflict resolution between parties of different age and rank."

"Interesting," many would comment. "And where's your office?"

"Oh," she replied. "My base of operation is my own home, and my best client is the Hanson Family Corporation."

One woman was so impressed, she told Kate, "I'd give anything to have a job like yours. And here I thought you were just a housewife!"

Charm is deceptive, and beauty does not last; but a woman who fears the Lord will be greatly praised. Reward her for all she has done. Let her deeds publicly declare her praise. —Proverbs 31:30, 31, NLT

The Importance of Goals

What if Sir Edmund Hillary had said, "I doubt if we can make it to the top of Mount Everest"? His name would have never made the *Guinness Book of World Records*.

What if Beethoven had said, "Whoever heard of a deaf composer?" and quit writing music? We'd be deprived of the beautiful strains of his ninth symphony!

What if the apostle Paul had lamented, "Now that I'm in prison, I'm too cold and stiff to write any letters"? A portion of the New Testament would never have been written.

Why did these individuals accomplish so much? Because they had goals.

When your children balk at practicing the piano or would rather watch Monday night football than tackle their homework, it's probably because they don't have goals.

Goals give a focus to life. As Edison once said, "Genius is one percent inspiration and ninety-nine percent perspiration." Without goals, the perspiration just isn't there!

Finishing is better than starting. Patience is better than pride. —Ecclesiastes 7:8, NLT

DR. KAY KUZMA

Developing Trustworthy Children

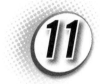

Make sure you and your maturing children agree on reasonable limits and the consequences for disobedience. Children usually don't mind proving their trustworthiness if they know they'll get more privileges because of it.

Trust is earned by keeping within the boundaries, such as being home at a certain time, reporting where they're going and what they'll be doing, and being there when they say they will be.

Don't be paranoid. Overprotective parents either smother their children's initiative or cause their kids to rebel. Give a little slack in your apron strings. How your children deal with the slack—the decisions they make in the gray areas—is what will build their sense of personal value and independence.

Chances are, you learned some of your most valuable lessons as a child through consequences. Good decision makers are developed by suffering the consequences of bad decisions. Don't bail children out too quickly if they make mistakes. Just make sure they know that you love them supremely, no matter what!

"If you know these things, blessed are you if you do them." —John 13:17, NKJV

Lessons From 409

Have you ever wondered why the cleaning product 409 was named 409? It's a very strange name, isn't it? I can understand why Fantastik is called Fantastik, and Mr. Clean makes sense. But 409?

Look closely at the label and you'll discover a possible reason for the name. In small letters above the big 409 is the word *formula*. Could it be that the producers had a goal to develop a cleaning product that was superior? Could it be they tried 408 formulas before they were satisfied?

What if they would have stopped at formula 408 and said, "It's impossible"? We would have all had to use another cleaning product!

When you or your children are tempted to say, "It can't be done; it's impossible," grab a bottle of 409, pray for persistence, and keep trying! Chances are, success is right around the corner.

"With men it is impossible, but not with God; for with God all things are possible." —Mark 10:27, NKJV

DR. KAY KUZMA

The Reconciliations Rug

One rather strong-willed couple knew that their marriage was headed for trouble if they weren't willing to make up quickly after a conflict.

They agreed that whenever they had an argument, the first one to step on what they called their "reconciliation rug," wanting to reconcile, would be the least guilty.

When tempers became heated, suddenly one would remember the rug. Each raced to reach the rug first, because each knew the other was more guilty! By the time they were standing on the rug, they were laughing, hugging each other, and ready to forgive.

I like the idea of a "reconciliation rug," especially if your kids are prone to bickering and squabbling with each other—and wanting their own way. Everyone makes mistakes. But being willing to say "I'm sorry" and "You're forgiven" can heal hurt feelings and restore peace.

If it takes a "reconciliation rug" to remind your family of the importance of forgiveness, perhaps you ought to have one in every room of the house!

"Your heavenly Father will forgive you if you forgive those who sin against you; but if you refuse to forgive them, he will not forgive you." —Matthew 6:14, 15, TLB

Nagging Ninny

A woman wrote to me saying her husband and children complained about her nagging. She'd tried to stop—but it had become a habit.

Here's what I advised, "The problem isn't yours; it's theirs! If they would just do what they are supposed to do, or do it the first time you asked, you wouldn't have to nag. Right?"

Here's the cure. Your family must retrain you to never make a request more than once. Here's how:

First, they must respond *immediately* when you ask them to do something.

Second, if they can't, they need to establish *when* you need the task completed.

Third, they should do it *without a reminder*.

Your family can't possibly lose. Sooner or later, they'll end up doing what you ask anyway. By responding immediately, they won't have to live with a nagging ninny, and your problem will be solved!

A nagging wife annoys like constant dripping. —Proverbs 19:13, TLB

DR. KAY KUZMA

Responsibility Versus Ownership

When you have a baby, it's easy to think, *This baby belongs to me.* But that's not true.
You are responsible to feed, diaper, bathe, entertain, educate, and pay for an incredible number of child-generated bills. But don't let responsibility be confused with ownership.

If you own something, it's yours to treat according to how you feel. The problem is, sometimes your feelings aren't too good! Parents who feel their children are objects they own, suffer tremendous guilt when children rebel; inflated pride when they succeed; and a deep sense of loss when they leave home.

If, however, you view your children as gifts on loan from God, you will parent from a different perspective. You'll monitor your words and actions so you won't be abusive. You'll want to fulfill your responsibility to train up God's children with Christlike love and discipline.

So before you act, ask yourself, "How would Jesus handle this?" because the child you're raising actually belongs to Him.

How great is the love the Father has lavished on us, that we should be called children of God! —1 John 3:1, NIV

Screaming Is Demeaning

Nobody likes to be screamed at—and it's especially damaging to children. Yet it happens so easily when we become frustrated, tired, and angry.

Shelley didn't scream very often, but when she saw her children having a mud fight in their good clothes, she lost her cool, ran to the door, and started to scream, "Kids!"

Suddenly, she noticed her neighbor planting flowers by the fence and was embarrassed. She didn't want him to know she sometimes lost her temper and screamed at her children, so she changed to a song, "Kids, would you come into the house today, would you come into the house today . . ."

Well, if you're in danger of losing your cool and damaging your child's self-worth—or your husband's or wife's—hopefully, you'll start screaming in the right key, so you can break forth in song and not hurt those you love.

I'd much rather have someone sing to me than scream—wouldn't you?

The tongue is a small thing, but what enormous damage it can do. A great forest can be set on fire by one tiny spark. And the tongue is a flame of fire. —James 3:5, 6, TLB

DR. KAY KUZMA

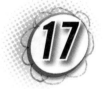

Children Are Like Apples

A pples remind me of children. They come in all shapes and sizes—and in many different colors and flavors. And yet, no matter how different apples look on the outside, there is something special on the inside.

Cut an apple through the middle—right through the equator—and you'll make the most wonderful discovery; you'll find a star that symbolizes something very special.

For just as every apple, no matter how different it is on the outside, has a star within its core, so does every child.

It's all there, just waiting to be discovered and nurtured. That's what parents are for—seeing the hidden potential of every child, encouraging those special talents to grow, and opening doors of opportunity so that the star of potential can shine.

Why don't you take time today to discover your child's star of potential?

Do not neglect the gift that is in you. —1 Timothy 4:14, NKJV

Option Living

Does your child sometimes feel like a misfit—doesn't like school and feels he or she can't do anything right? If so, option living is what is needed.

Option living means there are no roadblocks in life. No dead ends. No failures. Only possibilities.

If things aren't going well, don't let your child get sucked into the quicksand of overwhelming competition.

Your child is unique. Not everyone has to be tops in school or be a concert violinist. Don't force your ideals on your child. Look for other options that may better suit your child's God-given talents.

Why do we think every child has to take piano lessons or play in Little League or grow up to be a doctor, lawyer, or scientist? And why is it when he or she fails, we think the world has ended, instead of accepting this as an indication that the search for possibilities is still in progress?

Your child is special. Make sure he or she has enough options to keep feeling that way!

"Is anything too hard for the LORD?" —Genesis 18:14, NKJV

DR. KAY KUZMA

Catering to Children's Food Likes

What do you do with a child who won't eat anything but hot dogs and macaroni and cheese? Unless you like the idea of running a cafeteria, don't try to meet every family member's food likes at each meal.

Instead, have a family policy that everyone taste at least one bite of every dish. It can be a quarter of a teaspoonful, but at least it's a taste. Encourage them by saying, "Who knows, today may be the day your taste buds will change and you will like it!" Children who grow up with this policy do acquire a wider range of food likes.

If your child doesn't like what you are serving the family and has tasted her one bite, let her get her own meal. But limit the choice to healthful foods. Hot dogs and macaroni don't provide the variety of nutrients needed for healthy development and a strong immune system.

Don't make a big deal over finicky eaters. Food preferences change. Sometime in the future you may even hear, "Mom, please pass the asparagus."

[The Lord] satisfies your mouth with good things, so that your youth is renewed like the eagle's. —Psalm 103:5, NKJV

The Right-Brained Child

Do you enjoy learning facts, memorizing lists, and systematically solving problems? If so, you're probably left-brained. That means the left hemisphere of your brain is dominant. If you learn better from pictures, concrete objects, and direct involvement, then chances are, you're right-brained.

By the time we reach adulthood, most of us have learned to cope with how we learn best and can get along pretty well.

Getting good grades, however, can be a real problem for right-brained children, especially if they have left-brained teachers who provide a lot of work sheets and highly structured lessons. While left-brained children tend to do well with these activities, the creative right-brain learners struggle. Even though they may be smart, they often fail and end up becoming behavior problems.

So instead of trying to change the kids, maybe we as parents and teachers need to do a little changing ourselves.

"I applied my heart to know, to search and seek out wisdom and the reason of things." —Ecclesiastes 7:25, NKJV

DR. KAY KUZMA

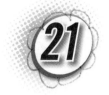

Reaching for the Stars

Parents want their children to aim high, yet not become discouraged with failure. The secret of success is to think of ideals as stars. They're easy to look at, tempting to wish for, difficult to reach, but essential for getting where you want to go.

Encourage your children to reach their ideals by setting realistic long-term goals. Then teach them to break each goal into manageable pieces—reasonable short-term objectives. Each objective reached brings your children one step nearer to success.

But they shouldn't try to reach the whole galaxy at once. It's easy to become discouraged or do a second-rate job when they attempt too much.

Tell your child, "Ideals are like stars. You may never reach them. But you can set your course by them. And when you do, you'll find yourself doing more than you ever thought possible."

I press on to reach the end of the race and receive the heavenly prize for which God, through Christ Jesus, is calling us.
—Philippians 3:14, NLT

Limits

Do you know the definition of *limit*? It's the point beyond which you are forbidden to go without suffering a consequence.

Have you ever wondered why children so often test or ignore the limits? The answer is that kids are pretty much like adults when it comes to obeying limits. Just ask some adults if they know what a speed limit is—and whether they have ever exceeded it.

They will answer, "Everyone goes over the speed limit occasionally. Besides, you never get a ticket for slightly going over the limit."

Then ask, "Would you go over the limit if you knew your car would explode?"

"No, of course not!"

Children ignore limits for the same reasons parents do. If the limit is unclear; if everyone's doing it; or if there's seldom a consequence, they'll take their chances.

Here's what you can do to encourage greater compliance: Make sure your limits are clear and specific. Then consistently enforce every limit with a significant consequence. And when kids obey, let them know how pleased you are.

Put these suggestions into practice, and your children will learn that you mean what you say and will be much more likely to stay within the limits.

The law of the LORD is perfect. —Psalm 19:7, NKJV

DR. KAY KUZMA

Slow as Molasses

Does it take your child hours to do something that would take you only a few minutes? Instead of getting upset, consider the following:

1. A child's concept of time is not the same as an adult's. An hour to you might seem like only a few minutes to your child. Or if waiting for Christmas—for a child a few days may seem like eternity.

2. You and your child may be programmed for different speeds, and you'll just have to accept this fact. Some people are low-gear people, while others speed around in high!

3. There may be too many distractions between your request and the place where it must be carried out. Put a TV set between the breakfast table and the bathroom sink, and it may take thirty minutes to get those teeth brushed!

4. Finally, a child may be purposely moving at a snail's pace to annoy you or get your attention. In this case, defuse your child's hidden anger with some active listening, and start building rapport and encouraging cooperation.

Young people, it's wonderful to be young! Enjoy every minute of it! —Ecclesiastes 11:9, NLT

Every Child Needs Irrational Love

Being irrational isn't usually something good. But I've discovered that when it comes to the kind of love that makes it possible for a child to grow up with a healthy outlook on life and a positive self-concept, the more irrational the love, the better.

In fact, I'd go so far as to say that children need at least one significant person in their lives who loves them irrationally—for no reason at all, other than that they exist. When parental love isn't tied to beauty, talent, or brains, *kids know they are truly loved*!

Ideally, your children know that you love them irrationally. In order to make sure they catch this unconditional love message, don't say things such as, "Daddy loves a good girl," or "I love you when you obey." You want your children to know that their behavior makes you happy, but it's not the reason you love them. Otherwise, children will feel that their parents won't love them if they are not good.

So when it comes to love, let it be irrational!

"For God so loved the world that he gave his only begotten Son." —John 3:16, KJV

DR. KAY KUZMA

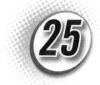

The Therapeutic Cry

Seeing someone cry usually makes us feel uncomfortable. Our first reaction, even with babies, is to try to stop the crying. What about parents? They aren't supposed to cry, are they?

Let's say, a crisis hits. You learn your wife has a terminal disease, your boy was crushed in a motorcycle accident, or your parents divorce. You scream, "It can't be happening!" and an overwhelming grief, anger, or pain settles in.

What should you do?

Send the kids next door to play or let them visit relatives so you can have some private time to cry—and cry hard. Mourn your loss. A therapeutic cry means you must empty your bucket of tears by crying so long that you haven't another tear to shed. It's only then that you can begin filling the void with something positive.

Between your therapeutic cries, allow God to comfort you, think positive thoughts, be compassionate to others, and, before long, you'll find the pain is not as intense.

Just as it takes time to mend a broken arm, it takes time to mend a broken spirit. So, don't be afraid to cry. It helps the healing.

You have collected all my tears and preserved them in your bottle! You have recorded every one in your book.
—Psalm 56:8, TLB

Let Children Bring Out Your Best

I remember when I first held my newborn. I thought, *How could this precious baby ever do anything wrong?* I was sure she would never sass, throw food, or scribble on the walls.

I also remember thinking what a great mom I was going to be. I was never going to spank or lose my cool. I would never get angry, yell, or criticize. Instead, I'd be patient and kind and handle discipline problems with creativity.

What happened to my ideal of being a perfect parent with perfect kids? It was destroyed by the real world of twenty-four-hour-a-day parenting. But in the process I've grown as a person. I've become much more understanding and accepting. Parenting has a way of doing that for you.

I hope you're having the same experience. Children can bring out either the worst in you—or the best. For your children's sake, make sure it's the best!

Above all these things put on love, which is the bond of perfection. —Colossians 3:14, NKJV

DR. KAY KUZMA

Letter Writing

Did you know that Abigail Van Buren, known to most as "Dear Abby," wrote her parents daily from the time she left home as a young girl until her parents' death! Those letters meant so much to them that they saved every one.

Telephone calls are wonderful. It's great to hear the other person's voice and speak of current interests. But calls are over so soon and you have nothing but the memory—and sometimes that's fuzzy. A letter you can read over and over—and relish each precious word. E-mailing is a great way to communicate—but there is nothing quite as special as a handwritten note.

Letters are great for long-distance communication, but they can also be meaningful to those you live with—especially when it comes to sharing your feelings or giving advice in a thoughtful way. A child who may not be interested in listening to what you have to say will often read the message. The best letter, however, is one filled with words of encouragement and appreciation.

Why not write a letter to someone in your family today?

Have I not written thirty sayings for you, sayings of counsel and knowledge? —Proverbs 22:20, NIV

The Empty Birthday Present Consequence

When kids do something wrong, too often parents lecture or punish. But there is a better way.

One time when my children were preschoolers, they decided to buy their daddy a box of his favorite candy for his birthday.

I put the box up on the top shelf of the pantry until I had time to wrap it. What I didn't know was that the children helped themselves to "Daddy's candy," and by the time I wrapped it, the box was empty.

"We can't give that present to Daddy," gasped the children.

"Why not?" I asked.

"Because it's empty."

There wasn't time to buy a new present, so they had to give their daddy an empty birthday present. They hung their heads in embarrassment when he opened it and had to explain they ate it all themselves.

I could have lectured them, but saying nothing and just allowing the natural consequence to happen was probably the best lesson of all! It never happened again.

The wages of sin is death, but the gift of God is eternal life in Christ Jesus our Lord. —Romans 6:23, NKJV

DR. KAY KUZMA

Why Children Misbehave

Children need positive attention. Criticism and negative comments are discouraging and often result in more misbehavior. But encouragement, optimism, and positive strokes are to kids like fertilizer is to plants. It's the stuff that really makes them flourish.

I know it may be hard for you to accept this. All your life you thought that when a child was misbehaving, he needed to be corrected. Well, that's true—but it must be balanced with enough positive encouragement so the child doesn't become discouraged and end up misbehaving even more.

Rudolf Dreikurs, a highly respected child psychiatrist, said, "Encouragement is more important than any other aspect of child-raising. It is so important that the lack of it can be considered the basic cause for misbehavior. A misbehaving child is a discouraged child."

I can't think of a better time than right now to seek out your child and administer a heaping dose of encouragement.

I delight to do Your will, O my God, and Your law is within my heart. —Psalm 40:8, NKJV

Answered Prayer

There is nothing like an answered prayer to increase a family's faith in God.

We had just climbed to the top of a twelve-thousand-foot-high mountain, when a child in our group began gasping for air and couldn't stand. We suggested he rest until he got used to the height. Then we prayed.

Soon a man arrived and said, "The child has altitude sickness. You've got to get him off the mountain immediately, or he could die!"

We took a quick but unfamiliar route down the mountain, and the child's altitude sickness disappeared. But so did the sun, and we were lost in the darkness, surrounded by rushing streams. We prayed for God's deliverance again.

Suddenly, a lone camper appeared and led us to the main trail.

Now when I look at Mount San Gorgonio, I don't just see a mountain. Instead, I see the two "angels" God sent to help us when we were in need.

Miracles are faith builders. I hope you're sharing with your family how God is daily working miracles in your life.

 The angel of the LORD encamps all around those who fear Him, and delivers them. —Psalm 34:7, NKJV

DR. KAY KUZMA

Catching the Positive

One day I took my daughters to Los Angeles for a shopping spree. I wasn't paying attention and parked in a zone marked "No Parking." When we returned, a ticket for fifty dollars was on the windshield. My heart sank. All that money thrown away on a senseless parking ticket!

I was tempted to grumble and gripe and make excuses. Then I thought, *Why let a silly mistake ruin the special time we had looked forward to for months?*

"Well," I said cheerfully, "I guess that's a lesson for me to read signs a little more carefully. At least I didn't park in a handicap zone. That fine would have been more than a hundred dollars!"

I want to be a positive person! I can either grumble when bad things happen, which accomplishes nothing except making myself and others miserable, or I can get on with the business of doing what I can to brighten my little corner of the world.

We know that all things work together for good to those who love God,
to those who are the called according to His purpose. —Romans 8:28, NKJV

Finding Something That Excites Your Child

Chris loved recess. But when it came to English, history, or math he would get sleepy, his eyes would water, and his mind would go riding waves or shooting baskets! And the result? Chris's parents hit the ceiling every time he brought his report card home!

Chris felt like a failure. But he wasn't. He had more creativity going for him than many entire classrooms of kids, but it wasn't being utilized until his mom brought home Barney Bump, a dummy—a ventriloquist doll.

Chris was thrilled. Immediately, his eyes brightened and he experienced a surge of motivational energy.

Every child needs to feel successful in something. Success breeds success. I have a feeling it won't be long before Chris's feelings of success as a ventriloquist might even have an impact on his grades.

Don't let your child feel like a failure. Search for those unique opportunities that will open doors of success and turn your child on to life!

I wish that all men were even as I myself. But each one has his own gift from God, one in this manner and another in that. —1 Corinthians 7:7, NKJV

DR. KAY KUZMA

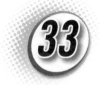

Childhood Perceptions of God

In a study of more than ten thousand children in the fifth through ninth grades, it was found that how children perceive God is associated with certain behaviors.

If children see God as a liberating God, who accepts them just as they are and loves them and forgives them, this correlates positively with high self-esteem, moral internalization, acceptance of traditional standards, achievement motivation, a positive attitude toward church, and pro-social behavior.

If children see God as restrictive, as stressing limits, controls, guidelines, and discipline, this view correlates with low self-esteem, sexism, racial prejudice, drug and alcohol abuse, and antisocial behavior.

The question is, Where do children pick up their perceptions of God?

From their parents.

What are you doing to help your children see God as a God who is liberal in love and forgiveness?

Behold what manner of love the Father has bestowed on us,
that we should be called children of God! —1 John 3:1, NKJV

Superglue Your Family

Most parents look forward to the birth of a child and are eager to cuddle, kiss, and coo to their new little namesake. But while getting bonded at birth is vitally important, too many parents have the mistaken idea that "once bonded—always bonded."

If you want your bonding birth experience to last a lifetime, you've got to "superglue" your family relationships by spending good times together on a regular basis. And there is no better way than through planning and celebrating family traditions—especially weekly or monthly ones.

Here are some suggestions: Have a monthly "picnic" in the living room; visit the zoo; go bowling; have Saturday pizza night. A tradition doesn't need to be expensive, but it should be regular so the kids can look forward to it.

Celebrating family traditions will make it easier for you to stay close to your children. I think you'll find that establishing traditions is a "superglue" experience!

Unless the Lord builds a house, the work of the builders is wasted. —Psalm 127:1, NLT

DR. KAY KUZMA

Meeting Children's Needs

A destructive myth is floating around the nooks and crannies of our homes. This myth states that parents ought to be able to meet all the needs of their children without any outside help.

Well, that just isn't true. The best parents are those with a wide circle of friends and relatives who help meet the children's needs and teach them important lessons.

One mother realized this when she caught her son with someone else's toy car hidden in his pocket. After they talked very seriously and he returned it, she assumed the lesson was learned. But after another "lost" item was found in his pocket, she called his teacher and asked her to kindly and privately confront him. The teacher did, and the lesson stuck.

Welcome help from others who are able to teach your children valuable lessons that they may have a difficult time learning from just you alone.

My God shall supply all your need according to His riches in glory by Christ Jesus. —Philippians 4:19, NKJV

36

A Date With Dad

I t takes time to establish good relationships with your children. Have you spent time one on one with each of your children lately? Perhaps you could borrow a good idea from my friend Lee.

When his children were just preschoolers, he began a monthly tradition of going on a "date" with each child. That first month, the kids were so eager that they argued over who would get to be Daddy's first date!

The evening usually started out by getting something special to eat, such as tacos or pizza. Whether they ended up watching goldfish and puppies at the pet shop or playing a round of miniature golf, spending time with Daddy was definitely a "cloud nine" experience.

When you spend quality time with your children, you are saying to them, "Hey, you are important to me!" Why don't you start planning a regular "date" with each of your children today?

The glory of children is their father. —Proverbs 17:6, NKJV

not for Kevin's father's Day

DR. KAY KUZMA

Love Notes

Are you an impulsive person? I hope so, because I have a marvelous idea of something you can do within the next five minutes that will bring a sparkle of excitement to your family!

Stop whatever you're doing, and pick up a pencil and paper. Now, write a love note to someone in your family. Everyone loves to receive them.

When my son was in the first grade, I had to drop by his school to visit the principal. While there, I wrote my son a little note and had it delivered by a classmate. I scribbled, "Dear Kevin, I love you. Love, Mom," and drew a big smiley face.

After school I asked Kevin if he received the note. "Oh yes, Mom," he said, "and everyone else at school wants one too!"

So why not be impulsive? Write love notes to your children, and they will put extra sparkles into their day—and yours as well!

"It is more blessed to give than to receive." —Acts 20:35, NKJV

Doing It for the Lord

What do you do when you really detest a task? Throw up your hands and refuse, or grumble and complain? Well, there's a better way!

Let me tell you about Denise, who hated doing the dishes. Her husband and three children dirtied dishes faster than she could wash them. At first she grumbled through the chore. Then one morning, she asked the Lord to change her attitude. And just like that, Ephesians 6:7 (NKJV) popped into her head: *"With good will doing service, as to the Lord, and not to men."*

As soon as she began visualizing her kitchen as God's kitchen—beautiful and spacious, with pearl bubbles and golden plates—her attitude about doing dishes changed. What an honor to be considered worthy of washing God's dishes!

 When you're faced with chores you dislike, why not do the task as if you're doing it for God Himself—and see it as an honor rather than a chore.

With good will doing service, as to the Lord, and not to men, knowing that whatever good anyone does, he will receive the same from the Lord. —Ephesians 6:7, 8, NKJV

DR. KAY KUZMA

The Power of Encouragement

Encouragement can change negative behavior. For example, a number of years ago we began noticing that the sunshine and laughter had disappeared from our little Kari. Her negative attitude was difficult to live with. After realizing that our interactions with Kari were constantly critical, especially my husband's, he decided to become her advocate to support and encourage her through difficulties rather than punish her.

Kari never knew anything about our plan, but within two days she was dancing circles around her daddy. "Oh, Daddy, I love you so much." Our little "grouch" had disappeared, and we were once more blessed with the warmth of her laughter.

What made the difference? Our encouragement and acceptance gave her a new sense of hope and enough "oomph" to discipline herself. Instead of negatively reacting to our criticism, she now responded in love to our encouragement.

Your right hand has held me up, Your gentleness has made me great. You enlarged my path under me,
so that my feet did not slip. —Psalm 18:35, 36, NKJV

Celebrating Anniversaries

Our three children really surprised my husband, Jan, and me on our eighteenth wedding anniversary. Just as we were leaving to go out for dinner, our twelve-year-old gave us a note and told us not to read it until we were driving.

We got into the car, waved goodbye, and started down the street. But the most awful racket was following us! Yes! It was the sound of aluminum cans tied to the back of the car!

Then I saw the sign our kids had put in the back window: "18th Wedding Anniversary."

I quickly unfolded the note. "Dear Mommy and Daddy: If you are embarrassed by the cans, the scissors are in the glove compartment."

Most people remember their tenth or twenty-fifth anniversary—but for us it's the eighteenth. It's amazing how a few cans and a little creativity can make an anniversary into an unforgettable experience.

A time to weep, and a time to laugh; a time to mourn, and a time to dance. —Ecclesiastes 3:4, NKJV

DR. KAY KUZMA

Dealing With Messy Kids

Do your children leave messes around the house that you finally pick up because you can't stand it any longer? If so, you're teaching your children that if they wait long enough, you'll do their work for them.

Here's a good rule to follow: *never do anything for children that they could benefit from by doing themselves.*

Make it a policy that messes must be cleaned up before bedtime. If you find a mess after your children have gone to sleep, wake them up and make them clean it up. Once or twice is all it takes to get the message across that you plan to enforce the policy.

Or you might let your children sleep and make sure the mess is cleaned up before breakfast time. Just remember, if you don't enforce the policy, your children won't take it seriously!

On rare occasions, if you clean up the mess, make sure your children know you've done it because you love them. Hopefully, they'll learn by imitation. *Hopefully!*

We love Him because He first loved us. —1 John 4:19, NKJV

God's Unlimited Resources

My brother hated mowing the lawn with our old push mower. Then one day he discovered a new resource. Friends! He knew Mom wouldn't let him pitch for the baseball team until the lawn was mowed, so he asked his buddies to bring over their lawn mowers for a lawn-mowing party. They ended up laughing and chasing each other around the yard until all the grass was cut. Then they happily grabbed their mitts and headed for the ball field. Working together certainly lightens the load, whether you're a kid—or a parent.

Friends are a wonderful resource. With friends you're not alone. Friends can make work more fun, and you learn to cooperate. So instead of giving up when faced with a big project, call in your friends—many hands do lighten the load.

And remember, God has resources that are beyond our wildest imagination. There is never a problem so big that it can't be solved.

Two are better than one, because they have a good reward for their labor. For if they fall,
one will lift up his companion. —Ecclesiastes 4:9, 10, NKJV

DR. KAY KUZMA

Why Kids Cheat

The chances are quite high that your children will cheat if the circumstances are right! What are the right circumstances for cheating?

1. When a number of other kids cheat, especially highly admired ones.
2. When your children's scores are common knowledge and their statuses in the classroom are determined by grade-point average.
3. When your children think there is no possibility they'll get caught.
4. If the rewards for cheating are so high that it's worth the risk.
5. If your children have a high internal need to be the best and will do anything necessary to attain this position.

Don't wait until the principal calls to tell you that your child has been suspended for cheating. Warn your children to be aware of the circumstances that will tempt them to cheat, and talk about what they should do to resist.

I hate every false way. —Psalm 119:128, NKJV

Dealing With Boredom?

Don't allow your children's complaints of boredom to make you feel guilty. It's not your responsibility to keep them entertained. It's their responsibility. Boredom is a cop-out. Boredom is an attitude problem.

Some children are bored when they are surrounded with the toys, games, and every imaginable trinket. Others can be completely absorbed with an old newspaper, crayons, and scissors. It's all in their minds!

So, if your children complain, "We're bored," toss the ball immediately back into their court, and ask, "What are you going to do about it?" Tell them they can either choose to be bored or choose to do something so they won't be bored. Don't feel you have to solve their boredom problem.

But to get them started, you could give them a stack of old newspapers and see how many things they can think of doing with them. Then give a prize to the most creative.

But we urge you, brethren, that you increase more and more; that you also aspire to lead a quiet life,
to mind your own business, and to work with your own hands, as we commanded you.
—1 Thessalonians 4:10, 11, NKJV

DR. KAY KUZMA

Can You Trust Your Kids?

Do you worry about what your increasingly independent kids are doing when they're out of your sight? Can they be trusted? Perhaps a more important question is, Can you trust their friends?

Regardless of how much you trust your own children, if they are running around with kids who do things you don't approve of, they'll probably yield to peer influence sooner or later.

Begin early to tell your children, "I can trust you only as much as I can trust your friends."

In addition, let them know that they have the power to influence their friends for good. Encourage them to be the "thermostat" that sets the moral temperature of their group, rather than the "thermometer" that measures the moral temperature.

Kids love freedom. It's surprising how responsible they can be if they know that the only way to get freedom is to prove to you that they are responsible and choose responsible friends.

And I will walk at liberty, for I seek Your precepts. —Psalm 119:45, NKJV

Goat-Getters

One of the fundamental laws of parenthood is, If children know what gets your goat, they'll get it. It's not that they want to persecute you. For the most part, children enjoy pleasing adults. But at times, children misbehave to get your attention, to win a power struggle, or just to reap the sweet taste of revenge. When children know what really upsets you, it gives them ammunition to get back at you when they're angry.

Typical "goat-getting" behaviors usually are things parents have very little control over, such as the kids saying dirty words, whining, lying, sassing, being lazy, or misbehaving when you're too busy to discipline. Undue attention to these behaviors is rewarding, and it's exactly what a child wants.

Therefore, react in a calm, matter-of-fact way. Be firm and impose a consequence, but don't dwell on the misbehavior. Don't let your kids know what really gets your goat!

Even a child is known by his actions, by whether his conduct is pure and right. —Proverbs 20:11, NIV

DR. KAY KUZMA

Taking Responsibility for Your Mistakes

Have you ever tried to squirm out of an uncomfortable spot by blaming others? It happened at the beginning of time. When Adam ate the forbidden fruit, he blamed Eve. And Eve? She blamed the serpent. Now, more than six thousand years later, we're still blaming others!

Just picture yourself in these common situations:

Company comes. You're behind schedule; the dishes aren't done, and things are all over the floor. You blame your kids, "If you would have helped me, this wouldn't have happened."

You receive a speeding ticket. Angrily, you turn to the children in the backseat, "Why didn't you get ready quicker? I wouldn't have had to drive so fast."

You leave the kitchen to answer the phone. When you return, the potatoes have burned. You say, "Kids, you were sitting right here. Why didn't you turn off the stove?"

It takes guts to own up to your mistakes, but your children will respect you if you do.

So the next time you goof, honestly say, "It's my fault. I'm sorry." You'll feel better about yourself when you take personal responsibility for what you do. And your kids will likely learn from your example.

And the LORD God said to the woman, "What is this you have done?" The woman said,
"The serpent deceived me, and I ate." —Genesis 3:13, NKJV

Brain Boosters for Bs and Above!

Grades aren't everything, but it sure does feel good to make an A on a tough exam. Your kids can do better on exams if they know how to study for maximum brain efficiency. Here's what you need to tell them:

The poorest position for learning is lying down. It's better to sit, but even better to stand. And if you really want to maximize your study time, walk! If you grip something in your hands, it will help. That's why the very best position is to walk while holding a book and turning pages.

Next, get rid of the clutter and distractions. You will learn material faster and better if you are able to focus. And taking a cat nap after a period of study will help your brain organize the material for better retention.

Finally, research shows that students who take an exam in the same room where they studied the material do better than those who don't. Why? Because objects in the room will trigger memory. So encourage your children to take advantage of class time to learn as much as possible!

Let our people also learn to maintain good works, to meet urgent needs, that they may not be unfruitful.
—Titus 3:14, NKJV

DR. KAY KUZMA

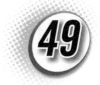

Dealing With Discouragement

Do you sometimes feel like the little cartoon character who was flying through the sky holding on to a helium-filled balloon?

"Things are pretty tough," he said, "when you're miles above the world holding onto a balloon."

In the next frame, he comments, "Of course, the balloon could pop—or I could be sucked into a jet stream . . ."

And the last frame says, "Isn't that the way it is in life. It never gets so bad but what it can't get worse."

Well, life as a parent is sometimes difficult—but there is always a solution!

When I begin to doubt it and need some encouragement, I open the book that never lets me down and start reading some of the promises I've underlined. It's amazing how much better I feel.

When you feel as if you're hanging on to a helium-filled balloon and life is getting you down, why don't you pick up your Bible—and take courage!

"Be strong and of good courage; do not be afraid, nor be dismayed,
*for the L*ORD *your God is with you wherever you go." —Joshua 1:9, NKJV*

Parents Can't Do Everything

Parents have a great influence on their children, but children are ultimately responsible for who they become. Perhaps you should start telling your child that

I gave you life, but I can't live it for you.

I can teach you things, but I can't make you learn.

I can buy you beautiful clothes, but I can't make you lovely inside.

I can offer you advice, but I can't accept it for you.

I can teach you to share, but I can't make you unselfish.

I can advise you about friends, but I can't choose them for you.

I can teach you about sex, but I can't keep you pure.

I can warn you about alcohol and other drugs, but I can't say No for you.

I can take you to church, but I can't make you believe.

I can tell you about lofty goals, but I can't achieve them for you.

I made some mistakes as a parent, but don't let them ruin your life. You can choose how you'll live, but my prayer is that, whatever you do, you'll do all to the glory of God.

Whether you eat or drink, or whatever you do, do all to the glory of God. —1 Corinthians 10:31, NKJV

DR. KAY KUZMA

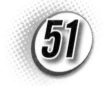

Are You on a Parental Seesaw?

Remember the seesaw on the playgrounds of your past? Too many parents play on a parental seesaw because they don't agree on how to discipline. Here's how it happens:

Let's say Dad comes home in a bad mood and demands, "Kids, why haven't the dogs been fed? And I told you before I left this morning that I wanted the leaves raked!"

What does Mom do? She will most likely go to the opposite extreme trying to balance Dad's authority with a little extra love.

Here's the problem: the more Dad leans to an extreme, the more it will force Mom to lean in the other direction—like a seesaw. Up-and-down. Back-and-forth. And eventually one moves too far back on the seesaw and falls off. Then *bang*—down crashes the other.

What kids really need is for their parents to get off the seesaw, move closer together in their parenting philosophies, and become more balanced in the way they deal with their children—with both parents being authoritative and both being loving.

"The Lord disciplines those he loves." —Hebrews 12:6, NIV

Teaching Children to Pray

Too often, praying is a ritual children perform at bedtime and before meals. What children really need is to learn how to talk with God all day long, not just when they need to say, "I'm sorry," "Please give me . . ." or "Thank You."

I doubt if you'd have many friends if you talked to them only when you'd done something wrong or when you needed something or you wanted to thank them. Relationships grow on chitchat, brainstorming, discussing ideas and plans, telling stories and jokes, sharing feelings, laughing and crying together.

Why not talk to God the same way?

One little girl, when asked if she'd said her prayers yet, replied, "Well, not exactly. I decided God must get pretty tired listening to the same old thing, so tonight I told Him the story of Goldilocks and the three bears."

Why not? I think God would be pleased if we shared something with Him we thought He'd really enjoy!

Oh come, let us worship and bow down; let us kneel before the Lord our Maker. For He is our God, and we are the people of His pasture, and the sheep of His hand. —Psalm 95:6, 7, NKJV

DR. KAY KUZMA

The Cushion of Love

Love is the protective agent that can soften the blow of psychological harshness or unfair discipline that sometimes comes from uptight, frustrated parents.

The thicker the cushion, the easier it is for the child to understand that parents will make an occasional mistake, without the child being devastated.

A loved child is much more likely to respond, "Dad sure got mad, but I know he didn't mean all those things he said," than a child who feels unloved.

Let's face it, if you're like me, you want to be a good parent, but you sometimes say things without thinking. Or maybe you threaten, criticize, or impose consequences that are too severe. I also hope you're learning from your mistakes, but because you're not yet perfect, I hope you've stored up a big cushion of love so your kids can bounce back without getting hurt.

"I have loved you with an everlasting love; I have drawn you with loving-kindness.
I will build you up again and you will be rebuilt." —Jeremiah 31:3, 4, NIV

Financial Independence Day

Charlie Shedd, a well-known author on the family, promised his newborn son, Peter, that by Peter's junior year in high school he could make his own financial decisions.

Wasn't that rather risky? How did he know Peter would turn out to be a financially responsible lad? And what made seventeen the magic year this was to happen?

Charlie didn't know for sure the exact date Peter would be ready for financial independence, but he did know that teenagers, whether ready or not, are going to make financial decisions.

Why not plan for that time and prepare your children? Why not set your children's financial independence day early enough so they can ask you for advice while they are still at home?

Good financial managers aren't born—they're developed.

"Where your treasure is, there your heart will be also." —Luke 12:34, NIV

DR. KAY KUZMA

From Nightmares to Sweet Dreams

If your children complain of having dreams that make them wake up shaking from fright, you need to monitor television, movies, comics, violent video games, and scary discussions about monsters in the closet and aliens in the attic. Children's imaginations run wild when fed on a diet of scary things. And it doesn't help to try to reason, "Dreams are make-believe," because if kids see it in their heads, it's real to them!

Instead, fill the hours before bedtime with pleasant activities. Read a fun bedtime story, sing songs, play table games, or put together a puzzle.

If the nightmares continue, add a night light and hang pictures of a guardian angel in their rooms to remind them of God's protection. Teach them to claim the promise of angel protection from Psalm 91:11.

Finally, talk about the dreams. Just the process of putting a dream into words makes it less scary. So take time to listen, reassure, and pray for sweet dreams.

He shall give His angels charge over you, to keep you in all your ways. —Psalm 91:11, NKJV

How Criticism Pops Balloons

"Can't you ever do anything right? You're going to be the death of me yet! What's wrong with you? Shape up or shut up!" Words of criticism can be incredibly cruel.

Think of your children as balloons blowing in the wind of everyday encounters. A balloon can take some pretty strong wind; it can be blown from one side to the other, but it won't pop. But let one tiny pin touch the balloon, and it explodes.

That's what criticism does to a child. It deflates the child's feelings of value and can destroy the will and zest for life.

Instead, encourage your children with words of appreciation, affirmation, encouragement, and praise. Catch them being good. Remind your children of times they succeeded in the past. Let them know you believe in them. Encouragement inflates balloons and allows them to soar; criticism pops them!

Do not let any unwholesome talk come out of your mouths, but only what is helpful for building others up according to their needs, that it may benefit those who listen. —Ephesians 4:29, NIV

DR. KAY KUZMA

Count Your Blessings

I t's an old familiar song. But the message is true.

> *Count your blessings, name them one by one*
> *And it will surprise you what the Lord hath done.*

So often we take our good days for granted, and as soon as a bad one comes along, we forget how much we have to be thankful for. And the more we count our troubles, the more our energy sags. Life seems hopeless.

Give yourself a shot of adrenaline. Start counting your blessings. In fact,

> *Count your blessings, name them two by two,*
> *And you will discover God's been good to you.*

A funny thing happens when you look back on the good things. You relive them and get to experience the joy all over again. The bad times in life are tough enough to live through the first time, so why recount them? Instead, relive the good, and you'll find yourself showered with more blessings.

"The LORD bless you and keep you; the LORD make His face shine upon you, and be gracious to you; the LORD lift up His countenance upon you, and give you peace." —Numbers 6:24–26, NKJV

58

Our Amazing Bodies

Our bodies are amazing! Did you know your heart beats about a hundred thousand times a day? And in every twenty-four-hour period, you breathe roughly twenty-three thousand times?

Isn't it amazing that your body maintains a steady temperature of 98.6 degrees under all weather conditions?

But there's more. To execute all your movements, you have more than seven hundred muscles. And you've been given more than seven million brain cells!

It's fascinating to me how wonderfully we have been made.

You know, if we could just purchase a new car with a tiny portion of all the incredible mechanisms that we find in our bodies, how carefully we would treat that car. We'd never put anything into the engine or fuel tank but the very best. Why then are we so careless about what we put into our bodies—and what we allow our children to put into theirs?

I praise you because I am fearfully and wonderfully made; your works are wonderful,
I know that full well. —Psalm 139:14, NIV

DR. KAY KUZMA

Character at Home

There's an old saying that goes, "Character is defined by what you are willing to do when the spotlight has been turned off, the applause has died down, and no one is around to give you credit."

Many parents are guilty of presenting their good sides to their business associates and friends, but when they walk in their front doors, they forget their company manners.

Are you a nice person at home? Are you fun to live with? Or do you let your defenses down and present a sagging character to those you love the best?

Benjamin Franklin thought his at-home character needed upgrading, so he chose thirteen character traits to work on, one a week for thirteen weeks. Then when the quarter ended, he started over again.

Why not try the same? Write down the thirteen most important character traits you would like to start working on. If you don't know where to begin, ask your children. Chances are they will have some excellent suggestions.

The righteous man walks in his integrity; his children are blessed after him. —Proverbs 20:7, NKJV

We Did It!

Have you ever played on a team where the superstar got all the attention—and credit—and you felt like a nobody? It isn't much fun, is it?

If you want your family to feel like a winning team, make sure that every family member feels like a superstar.

For more than a year, I had been working on a book manuscript. When it was almost finished, I got the crazy idea that the whole family should celebrate this accomplishment.

The day we mailed off the manuscript to the publisher, we headed to town to purchase five T-shirts that read, "WE DID IT!" with that day's date.

On special occasions when we all wore our "We Did It" shirts, the kids proudly explained to those who asked, "That was the day we finished writing a book."

Sometimes parents find themselves pushing for deadlines. When you do, let each member feel he or she is an important part of the project and celebrate when the project is completed.

Love each other with brotherly affection and take delight in honoring each other. —Romans 12:10, TLB

DR. KAY KUZMA

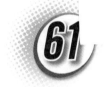

Quantity Versus Quality Time

Quality versus quantity is an age-old argument when it comes to spending time with children. Which is more important?

If you want to be an effective parent, the answer is, you had better be sure you give your children plenty of both!

Consider a morning when Mom shouts, "Come to breakfast!" and fumes when the milk is spilled. Then Dad yells, "Hurry up! You're going to make me late!"

This is time together, but it's certainly not quality time.

Where does quantity come in? According to a study conducted a number of years ago by family researcher Urie Bronfenbrenner, the typical father of a one-year-old spent on the average only 37.7 seconds per day with his infant.

If that's all the time you are spending with your child, there's no way you can pack in enough quality to have a meaningful relationship.

What's the answer to the quality-versus-quantity question? Make sure you give your children plenty of both!

---

*"Could you not watch with Me one hour? Watch and pray, lest you enter into temptation.
The spirit indeed is willing, but the flesh is weak." —Matthew 26:40, 41, NKJV*

From the Inside Out

Have you tried to be a good parent, but when the children get on your nerves, you end up losing it? Perhaps you're working on the wrong thing. The behavior you don't like in yourself might be caused by something inside, such as unhealed hurts of the past, resentment, and hidden anger.

It's like the worm in an apple. Have you ever wondered how it gets there? Believe it or not, I've been told it comes from the inside! An insect lays an egg in the blossom, and then after the apple has formed, the worm hatches and eats its way to the outside.

Many of our expressed negative emotions are like that. They come from the inside. The answer is to seek professional help to kill the worms of resentment and anger before they can eat their way into our behavior and destroy relationships and our homes.

"A good man out of the good treasure of his heart brings forth good things, and an evil man out of the evil treasure brings forth evil things." —Matthew 12:35, NKJV

DR. KAY KUZMA

Stop the Destruction of Families

I was shocked a number of years ago when I read that in every twenty-four-hour period
- 2,750 of America's children learn that their parents are divorcing.
- 1.3 million youngsters are latchkey kids.
- 500 children between the ages of ten and fourteen will start using drugs.
- 100 children will begin using alcohol.
- 90 children will be removed from their homes and will be placed in foster care.
- And 4 children will die from the effects of child abuse.

All that in just one twenty-four-hour day!

If only we could stop the clock—how many lives would be saved, how many marriages put back together, and how many children would have the opportunity to discover the joy and promise of what family should be!

Time, however, can't be stopped. But the destruction of families can. You can make a difference by recommitting yourself to your family, solving problems early, and getting professional help if needed.

Your wife shall be like a fruitful vine in the very heart of your house, your children like olive plants all around your table. Behold, thus shall the man be blessed who fears the LORD. —Psalm 128:3, 4, NKJV

The Reluctant Working Mother

Millions of mothers working at outside jobs would, if they had the choice, rather be home with their children. Debra was one of those moms who loved to be home, but when Tom lost his job, she had no choice. Here's how she managed with a full-time job:

First, she quit trying to be Supermom and budgeted her time for the housework, doing only those things that were absolutely necessary.

Next, Debra began counting her blessings. She was thankful that she was healthy enough to work and that she could get a job during a time of economic crisis. The kids were becoming much closer to their dad and were happy. She was making new friends. Plus, she even found herself planning more special activities for her family to do together.

Working may not be your first choice, but, like Debra, with a positive attitude and good planning, you can be a good mom and work outside the home too.

Nothing is better for a man than that he should eat and drink, and that his soul should enjoy good in his labor. This also, I saw, was from the hand of God. —Ecclesiastes 2:24, NKJV

DR. KAY KUZMA

Oatmeal on the Ceiling

Does this sound like your house?

> *There's oatmeal on the ceiling,*
> *And crumbs upon the floor.*
> *The windows all need washing*
> *And jam's spread on the door.*

If so, you're probably in the middle of parenting.

I don't believe you should live in a pigsty, but there is no way you're going to keep all the fingerprints off the walls if you're really enjoying your kids.

Far too many parents spend their precious time cleaning up after the kids, instead of playing with them, and eventually the kids grow up and leave you with a sterile house and few memories. I'd much rather have the memories of squat tag, butterfly kisses, and watching my kids feed the ducks, wouldn't you?

Major in your children, even though there may be "oatmeal on the ceiling," and I'll guarantee you'll never regret it.

Now he who plants and he who waters are one, and each one will receive his own reward according to his own labor.
—1 Corinthians 3:8, NKJV

Family Rivalry Versus Loyalty

Family loyalty is important. Siblings should not be allowed to treat each other in ways that are demeaning or that cause self-worth to be destroyed. Instead, they should be encouraged to support and help each other.

Name-calling and tattling are often beginning signs of sibling rivalry. If your home has become a verbal battlefield, carefully analyze your family's life to determine what might be causing this rivalry. There could be some underlying jealousy that needs to be healed before the war can be won.

Check to see if your local library has some children's books on jealousy. A story is a great way to introduce the topic. Then be willing to listen to feelings without taking sides or criticizing. You might get some valuable insights into what is causing the rivalry and what you may be unconsciously doing to contribute to it.

Getting rid of the cause will most likely get rid of the problem.

Whoever hates his brother is a murderer, and you know that no murderer has
eternal life abiding in him. —1 John 3:15, NKJV

DR. KAY KUZMA

Finding the Key for Self-Motivation

I could make a fortune if only I knew the magic formula for self-motivation. I do know children need to feel good about themselves. Where do they shine? What are their interests? Many times, finding success in one area spills over into others.

And, of course, a challenging school environment helps—probably one where children can advance at their own rates, get immediate rewards and compete with self, not with others. The complaint of many unmotivated children is, "There's always someone better, so why should I try?"

The real key, however, is to find someone who can communicate these ideas to children: "You are special. I like you. You have so many talents. This work is easy-breezy; you can do it. You're one superbright kid. You can do anything you want to do." If you can change your children's negative self-perceptions, into positive ones, that "I can" spirit will take over and become the motivation necessary for success.

A desire accomplished is sweet to the soul. —Proverbs 13:19, NKJV

Levels of Communication

Most of the time we communicate in clichés. Without thinking, we say, "Hi, how are you?" "Nice day, isn't it?" But if mere chitchat is the main substance of your communication with your children, then there isn't much satisfaction.

How much better to at least report things that have happened to you or share facts that you have heard. No one can argue with a report, unless it's not reported accurately. You show you're interested in each other by reporting something you think they would like to hear—or need to hear.

But you'll learn more about each other if you'll talk about your ideas and opinions, which is the next higher level of communication. There is a risk involved, that your child will think differently about certain issues. But along with the risk, there is the added satisfaction of sharing what is on your heart.

Don't stop there. Real closeness comes when you share your feelings. Because they shape behavior, you'll find communicating with your child on the feeling level is the most meaningful of all.

Give ear to my prayer, O God, and do not hide Yourself from my supplication. —Psalm 55:1, NKJV

DR. KAY KUZMA

Resisting Peer Pressure

Have you ever heard your child say, "I can't wear that. The kids will laugh at me"? Well, either it's a legitimate worry, or children may be using that excuse to get what they want.

Establish bottom-line standards concerning morality, integrity, safety, and health that are so important that you will not give in to your children just because they think kids will laugh at them.

But hairstyles or the clothing they wear, as long as it's modest, shouldn't fall into this category.

On those things that do, your children must learn to stand against peer pressure. Talk about situations in which they may be tempted to compromise their standards, such as smoking or drinking alcohol, and role-play ways to say No.

Children who decide what is right and wrong and practice saying No before they face the temptation will be far better prepared to resist negative peer pressure than those who don't.

Do not enter the path of the wicked, and do not walk in the way of evil. Avoid it, do not travel on it; turn away from it and pass on. —Proverbs 4:14, 15, NKJV

Children Need You

The statistics are frightening. A few years ago, a United States report said approximately one million teenagers were either runaways or "latchkey" kids, who came and went without parental direction. UNICEF has suggested that there are more than one hundred million children in the world who are abandoned by their families and become street children.

You may not have a runaway, and you probably haven't abandoned your children, but just how involved are you? Do you know what they're doing after school? Do you know the names of their best friends? And do you take time to listen and encourage? How long has it been since you went someplace together?

Teenage suicide is up, and one of the factors seems to be the lack of meaning and direction in the teenagers' lives. Parents have high expectations for their children but fail to take the time to communicate how success can be achieved. When children need emotional support, many have no place to go.

Kids need direction—but above all, they need you!

"Can a woman forget her nursing child, and not have compassion on the son of her womb?
Surely they may forget, yet I will not forget you." —Isaiah 49:15, NKJV

DR. KAY KUZMA

When Life Begins

Three mothers were discussing when life begins. The first said, "Life begins at conception. In fact, did you know you can hear a baby's heartbeat at just eighteen days?"

The second listened but offered a different opinion. "No," she said, "life begins at birth. When you can cuddle your newborn, look into your baby's eyes, and nurse her. And when the baby smiles at you for the first time, now that's when life really begins."

The third mother, who was just a little older, shook her head. "Life begins," she said with conviction, "when the kids leave home—and the dog dies!"

I don't know what stage of life you're in. Maybe you're thinking about having children, actually expecting one, or rearing a dozen and dreaming about your emancipation day. But whatever stage it is, I hope you're living it to the fullest. Children grow up quickly. Enjoy them while you can.

Rejoice in the Lord always. Again I will say, rejoice. —Philippians 4:4, NKJV

How Are You Spending Your Time?

Parents can either choose to spend their time on things or on relationships. The temptation for most is to focus on things. When you've worked extra hours to buy a new car, people notice. Or if you spend your time dusting and picking things up, you can brag about a clean house. But if you spend that time pushing your child in a swing or shooting baskets with your teen, what do you have to show for it?

Housework and job responsibilities are never done. They can consume all your time because there's always more!

To make sure your children are your *first* priority, limit the time you're willing to give to things such as housework or making money. Instead, focus on the relationships you are building with your family by spending positive time together with them.

Martha was the jittery type, and was worrying over the big dinner she was preparing. She came to Jesus and said, "Sir, doesn't it seem unfair to you that my sister just sits here while I do all the work? Tell her to come and help me." But the Lord said to her, "Martha, dear friend, you are so upset over all these details! There is really only one thing worth being concerned about. Mary has discovered it—and I won't take it away from her!" —Luke 10:40–42, TLB

DR. KAY KUZMA

Role Model and Mentor

Regardless of what you do, you're going to have a tremendous influence on your children's lives. Your children are going to follow your example about how to act when they get frustrated or angry and about how to rejoice when something goes well.

They're going to learn to talk like you do. In all your daily interactions, you'll be teaching your children lessons that will affect the way they live their entire lives.

Children are not blank slates upon which we can write whatever we want. They're born with their own personalities and temperaments. But they are like sponges. Your children are absorbing everything about you.

You can't choose whether or not to influence your child. *You will influence them.* But you can choose whether your influence will be positive or negative.

Look at your life. Are you the kind of person you want your child to grow up to be? If not, you better make some changes quickly!

Avoid every kind of evil. —1 Thessalonians 5:22, NIV

Love Is What Families Are For

I once saw a bumper sticker of a pig happily sitting in the mud. The caption read, "To know me is to love me." My immediate reaction was that I could never love a pig! But then I thought, if I were given a little piglet as my very own, and if I slept with it, nursed it through illnesses, and saw it respond to my love and attention, I bet I *would* love it!

Now I don't want to suggest that our children are like pigs. But there's truth in the bumper sticker.

We all know that some children are easy to love, and others—well, loving them is a challenge.

Yet if we really get to know these difficult children, rock them to sleep, nurse them through illnesses, and watch them respond to our care and attention, and truly begin to understand them—we would grow to love them.

Love is what families are for.

We love Him because He first loved us. —1 John 4:19, NKJV

DR. KAY KUZMA

Name-Calling Is Dangerous

Children, especially young ones, take seriously the names they are called. If children are called a negative word, such as *stupid* or *dummy,* often enough, it becomes like a negative script that can affect their lives. They begin to think they are stupid or dumb.

Kids easily acquire the habit of calling people—especially their siblings—bad names when they are frustrated with them. That's why you must stop name-calling immediately. Calmly say, "You may not hurt another person, and calling people names hurts their feelings. If you children can't get along together, I will have to separate you two."

Children pick up name-calling from TV, friends, and occasionally from parents who mutter "idiot" or "crazy" when someone cuts in front of them on the freeway.

To retrain the entire family to see people in the most positive light possible, you might play this game: If someone calls someone else a bad name, they have to immediately say three positive things about that person. It can be fun—and educational too.

A fool vents all his feelings, but a wise man holds them back. —Proverbs 29:11, NKJV

Borrowing the Love You Don't Have

My friend Trish had in-laws who spent the winter months at her home because they wanted to enjoy the grandchildren. On the last day of their previous visit, Trish and her mother-in-law had a terrible argument, making it extremely difficult to communicate during the year. Trish dreaded having them come again.

The day the folks arrived for their long winter's stay, Trish was thinking, *If only I could borrow a little love; then maybe I wouldn't have so much hate. And then an answer came to her.* "Why not borrow some love from God?"

The idea intrigued her. She purchased a present and smiled as she gave it to her mother-in-law. *It's a love gift from God,* Trish thought to herself, but her mother-in-law thought it was from Trish. And the flowers and card left in their room weren't from Trish either, but the folks thought so.

The result was a sweet, cooperative mother-in-law. The two of them didn't always agree, but a little love—even though it was borrowed—sure made a difference.

"You have heard that it was said, 'You shall love your neighbor and hate your enemy.' But I say to you, Love your enemies and pray for those who persecute you." —Matthew 5:43, 44, RSV

DR. KAY KUZMA

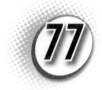

Unclutter Your Life

Do you feel pressured with too much to do? Are there too many toys to pick up? Too many things to read? Too many clothes to wash?

Well, I have a great idea of how you can be good to yourself. Unclutter your life! Get rid of the stuff you never use. Go through your closet and get rid of anything you haven't worn in a year.

Do you really need all those books? And what about those broken toys—or the ones your child has outgrown? And why are you saving the puzzle that has pieces missing? Recycle the plastic and glass containers. And throw away the pencil stubs.

Drop memberships in organizations in which participating has become an unpleasant chore. Cancel subscriptions to magazines you don't read. And if charities that you're not interested in keep writing to you, ask them to take your name off their mailing lists.

When you do, you'll have less to shuffle, pick up, put away, and sort through, and more time to enjoy yourself and your family.

Let all things be done decently and in order. —1 Corinthians 14:40, NKJV

Bitter or Better Over Parents' Mistakes

What do you do if your children are past the early years where character and personality are most easily influenced, and you haven't done such a great job of parenting?

You can't start over. But it's never too late to get the message across to them that they are loved supremely and unconditionally, even if there were times in your past when you didn't act like it!

Say, "I'm sorry for the mistakes I made," but don't let your children dump all the blame for their problems on you. Throw the ball back into their court with words like these: You may choose how the mistakes I made will affect your life. You can either grow bitter or better. I hope you will grow *better* by determining you won't make the same mistakes!

And when you begin to feel guilty, remember, if God can forgive you when you ask, shouldn't you forgive yourself?

For You, Lord, are good, and ready to forgive, and abundant in mercy to all those who call upon You.
—Psalm 86:5, NKJV

DR. KAY KUZMA

Shrinking Negative Emotions

Humans have become quite sophisticated in their ability to shrink things. We can take a filing cabinet full of documents and shrink them down so they can be stored on one tiny microfilm. And we've put more power into a laptop computer than was available in computers requiring giant rooms just a few decades ago. In fact, my little laptop has far more memory than the computers that sent men to the moon in the sixties.

There's one giant, however, that we're still struggling with. We think we have it conquered, and then our children get on our nerves, and we've lost control once again.

What's the uncontrollable giant? Emotions—especially those ugly ones that seem to grab us without warning and cause us to act irrationally.

We can't avoid them, but we can learn how to shrink them so they don't control us. We do this by recognizing the emotions early and dealing with the causes of the emotions before we are forced to act out our feelings in ways that hurt ourselves and our families.

You will keep him in perfect peace, whose mind is stayed on You, because he trusts in You.
—Isaiah 26:3, NKJV

Spontaneous Time

Do you spend time with your children on the spur of the moment? Or do you resent them for interrupting you? When my son Kevin was three, I was busy writing an article on the importance of spending quality time with children when he asked, "Mommy, can I help you type?"

I said, "Kevin, I'm very busy writing an important article, and I don't have time to let you type now." Dejected, Kevin retreated to the other room.

As I read over the last few sentences of my article, the light dawned—quality time together! That's what Kevin needed now, not later!

"OK, it's your turn," I called. As his fingers flew over the keyboard, I sat back to enjoy my son. But after three minutes, he hopped off my lap, said, "I'm finished," and disappeared. What Kevin wanted was not so much to type, but some love and attention from his mom!

The next time your child needs a little extra love and attention, why don't you welcome his or her interruption and enjoy some special time together?

It is senseless for you to work so hard from early morning until late at night, fearing you will starve to death; for God wants his loved ones to get their proper rest. Children are a gift from God; they are his reward.
—Psalm 127:2, 3, TLB

DR. KAY KUZMA

Don't Bend to Kid Pressure

Mom, I just have to have those jeans! Everybody's wearing them! And I gotta get those Air Jordans. Nobody wears these ugly, cheap things!"

If you are tempted to buy your children something because you can't stand the pressure, don't! By being firm and resisting their begging, you will teach them one of the most important lessons in life: *one does not have to bend to pressure.*

Perhaps the best way to resist yielding is making sure that they have their own checking accounts. The next time you hear those irresistible pleading voices asking for some expensive item, take a deep breath, smile, and say, "Yes, you can have it, if you have the money to pay for it."

If you want to buy your children something special, fine. Just don't do it after they pressure you. Otherwise, you are rewarding them for this bullying behavior, and it will likely get worse.

Blessed is the man who endures temptation; for when he has been approved, he will receive the crown of life which the Lord has promised to those who love Him. —James 1:12, NKJV

Take Time for Recommitment

I once had a mom ask, "How can I get control of my life? My three boys are constantly fighting, the baby is demanding, the house is a mess, and my husband is no help! I have to end up screaming to get anyone's attention!"

My advice was for her to spend more time with her husband.

"What? That's not fair," she cried. "The children need me, and he can take care of himself."

My reply was that after a hurricane, you don't worry about the shingles until you've shored up the foundation. Without a strong foundation, it won't be long and the shingles won't be needed. Then I explained that without a strong marriage, there was little hope that the children would survive unscathed.

"Why not make plans for a romantic weekend for two and recommit your lives to each other," I suggested. "With that commitment you can then begin working through your problems together. And you'll be much more likely to be successful."

She and her husband planned a fun weekend together and came home with renewed energy and some creative problem-solving ideas.

It's amazing how taking a little time away from the kids can give you a new perspective on life. Parents need that occasionally.

In everything you do, put God first, and he will direct you and crown your efforts with success.
—Proverbs 3:6, TLB

DR. KAY KUZMA

Cookies and Milk and a Listening Ear

I once met an eighty-seven-year-old woman who lived next door to two school-age children and across the street from three more. "I love these children," she said. "They visit me and call me Grandma, and I give them chocolate-chip cookies and milk. But I would like to do something more to show them they're loved."

I thought, *If only there were more older folks who felt like this dear lady. What a brighter place this world would be for children. And what a blessing for parents to have neighbors who love their kids.*

What more could this grandma do? A listening ear is the best gift anyone can give a child. The second thing is to share your value system. Tell character-building stories and model honesty, sympathy, and kindness.

Finally, I told her to keep on serving cookies and milk, because as the kids grow older and spend more time with their friends, they are likely to experience their share of rejection and failure. And when they do, I hope they will recall the cookies and milk and get a warm, fuzzy feeling knowing that they are loved not just by their parents, but others too.

When God's children are in need, you be the one to help them out. —Romans 12:13, TLB

Teach Kids to Stand Up to Bullies

Prepare your children to deal with threatening bullies. One meaningful way is to role-play the following situations:

They can call the child's bluff. "OK, go home. You can come back and play when you are ready to share."

They can negotiate. "If you really want the toy that badly, you can have the toy this time, but next time I get the first choice of what I want to play with."

They can stand up for their rights. "It's my toy. I can choose who plays with it."

They can share their feelings. "I don't like it when you always get your way. It makes me mad."

They can set standards. "One rule of this house is no threats. You will have to leave if you threaten me again."

Don't fight your children's battles for them. If you do, children think they are incapable of solving their own problems and will become even more dependent and vulnerable to peer abuse. Instead, teach them how to stand up for themselves.

The LORD is the strength of my life; of whom shall I be afraid? —Psalm 27:1, NKJV

DR. KAY KUZMA

Thumbs Down on Allowances

I don't believe in allowances! Parents who give their children money just because they exist are training them for welfare. Instead of fostering industriousness and hard work, this fosters irresponsibility.

Some kids persecute their parents with angry words: "I don't care what you think," or "You can't make me." And then at the end of the week, they pick up their allowance, thinking that their families owe it to them.

Love, discipline, lessons on spiritual values, and meeting basic needs are all things parents owe their children. Money isn't one of them.

Instead, an allowance should be conditional on the child acting responsibly, behaving appropriately, and doing chores around the house. When the conditions are met and the money is handed over, there should be no strings attached. The kids have "earned" their money and should have the responsibility to spend it, give it, or save it as they please.

"I am the LORD your God, who teaches you to profit, who leads you by the way you should go."
—Isaiah 48:17, NKJV.

Help Kids Beat the Winter Blahs

Just because it's stormy outside, doesn't mean you have to put up with stormy relationships inside. A little creativity can transform your children's winter blahs into a blast. Here are some ideas for a starter:

Declare a bathroom beach day. Heat up the bathroom, have the kids dress in bathing suits, and fill the tub with water toys. Get a good book to read as you watch them. Then have a picnic lunch on a blanket on the floor!

Build a tent city. Bring out the blankets, sheets, and clothespins and allow your kids to build tents over tables and chairs. Have a "camp fire" in the fireplace or use the flame on your gas stove and roast hot dogs.

Have a stuffed animal party. Your children can make invitations send them to all their stuffed animals, bake cookies, and then have a party by blowing bubbles and playing games. Then have the stuffed animals help with the cleanup!

And whatever you do, do it heartily, as to the Lord and not to men. —Colossians 3:23, NKJV

DR. KAY KUZMA

How to Solve Child-Rearing Differences

Disagreeing over how to raise a child can be a thorn in an otherwise rosy marriage, unless you follow these ten "commandments."

1. Resolve your differences as soon as they arise.
2. Promise to not disagree in front of the children.
3. Attend a parenting class together and discuss new methods of child rearing.
4. Read parenting books together.
5. Don't blindly follow your parents' methods.
6. Own up when you make mistakes with your children.
7. Bite your tongue when tempted to say, "I told you so."
8. Promise each other that if either one wants to go for family counseling, the other will also agree to go.
9. Establish ground rules for open communication.
10. Pray that God will give you an understanding heart and insight into how to "train up a child in the way he should go" (Proverbs 22:6, NKJV).

Teach a child to choose the right path, and when he is older, he will remain upon it.
—Proverbs 22:6, TLB

Learn to Confront, Not Abuse

It takes practice to learn how to confront someone and openly share your feelings in a way that can lead to a solution, rather than being verbally abusive. A family can role-play different situations and say different things to each other and have the rest of the family judge whether they are confronting constructively or abusing verbally.

For example, here's an abusive statement: "That was a dumb thing to do." And here's a confrontational one that doesn't put the other down: "It hurts my feelings to be screamed at."

Now what about this statement? "You're just a slave driver; you always command, 'Do this, or do that.' " The sentence is abusive because it casts blame on the other person.

A confrontational statement points out the problem without blaming or negatively labeling the other person. Usually beginning the sentence with the word *I* instead of the word *you* will avoid an abusive statement. "I don't like to be bossed around," is much better than, "You're bossy!"

Use constructive confrontation and stop verbal abuse.

"By your words you will be justified, and by your words you will be condemned."
—Matthew 12:37, NKJV

DR. KAY KUZMA

Too Much Too Soon Isn't Good

When does food taste the best, on an empty stomach or a full one? Of course, you enjoy eating most when you're hungry. And it's best to savor the taste of the food rather than gobbling it down.

It's the same with gifts and children. They will enjoy a gift most when they aren't inundated with things.

That's why we do our children a disservice on birthdays or Christmas when we surround them with a mountain of presents. They grab the biggest package, tear off the wrapping, open the box, take a look, and discard the gift in their rush to get to the next one. And in the end they are often disappointed and ask, "Is that all?"

Instead, the fewer the gifts, the better. Sprinkle them throughout the year rather than all at once. And don't rush the gift opening. Make a ceremony out of it. Let them open a gift while all are watching, and then take time to explore it and express thanks. Then give someone else a turn.

"It is more blessed to give than to receive." —Acts 20:35, NKJV

Internal Boiling Causes Explosions

Internal boiling will eventually cause explosions if there is no way to express those negative emotions. When children are angry, throw temper tantrums, and scream verbal threats, they're letting off steam. Believe it or not, this is healthy. If a volcano can let steam off a little at a time, the chance of a devastating eruption is lowered, and you're alerted to an underlying problem. It's the same with children.

But this doesn't mean you should ignore this behavior. Rather, look at these symptoms as early warning signals. Something isn't right, and an emergency plan needs to be implemented to prevent a major incident.

Be on the watch for the first signs that anger is building. Pay attention to body language, as well as the children's words, and solve the problem at that level.

If children's emotional needs are met early, they don't need to explode later.

"Do not let your anger burn." —Genesis 44:18, NKJV

DR. KAY KUZMA

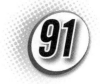

Preventive Therapy for Negativism

When your child tests you with out-of-bounds behavior, you may be tempted to correct every minor infraction, fearing that if you relax your restrictions, the behavior will get worse.

But the opposite may be true. A constant diet of "no, no, no," can cause a negative reaction, and the chances are quite likely that you'll end up getting more misbehavior.

Instead, start feeding your children a positive diet. Catch them being good. Smile. Wink. Let your children know that they are loved and that you like to be around them.

Don't bug them with a constant barrage of "Sit up straight, blow your nose, and don't talk with your mouth full." For the moment, you may have to ignore some of these things in order to build a more positive relationship with them. It will be easier for you to correct these behaviors when you're not "the enemy."

So, stop behavior that is absolutely forbidden, but spend the majority of your time on catching your children being good. It's great therapy for negativism!

Do not provoke your children to wrath. —Ephesians 6:4, NKJV

Boys and Guns

Gun play is typical play, especially among growing boys. I know. My boy had an obsession with guns—especially when he was playing with his friends. I never bought him a gun, because they looked too real and fostered "killing" games.

But somehow my son acquired a squirt gun. And he and his friends were always creative enough to come up with their own brand of weapons. Branches from trees became rifles. And I've put up with Lego guns, Tinker Toy guns, guns whittled out of soft wood, and crudely pounded and glued-together pieces of wood that became guns.

I've come to the conclusion that guns and boys go together—like jewelry and girls. The message: guns make boys feel strong and invincible, just like jewelry makes girls feel beautiful.

But to make sure children's play doesn't foster violence, you must set clear standards on how toy guns can be used. Toy guns are for pointing at targets, not at people.

All the nations will convert their weapons of war into implements of peace. —Isaiah 2:4, TLB

DR. KAY KUZMA

Tucking in Your Kids Long Distance

Many dads and moms can't be home to tuck their little ones into bed—the trucker out on the road, the on-call physician, the second-shift factory worker, the traveling sales rep, or the pastor holding evening meetings. You'd like to be home, but it's impossible.

Well, here's a great long distance way to tuck your kids in. Make an audio- or video-recorded message and say something like this: "Daddy can't be there right now, but I love you very much. And if I were there, I'd tickle your toes and give you a big bear hug and a butterfly kiss. But right now, grab yourself and give yourself a hug from me and get ready to catch the kiss I'm blowing to you. Did you catch it?" Then tell them a bedtime story and close with prayer.

Or if your child's bedtime comes at a time when you can take a break, just give them a call. With an Internet connection you might even Skype them or use your smart phone so they can actually see you.

The sound of your voice—or even seeing you long distance—isn't as good as being together, but it does bring children a sense of security knowing that they're loved regardless of where you are.

"Therefore you now have sorrow; but I will see you again and your heart will rejoice, and your joy no one will take from you." —John 16:22, NKJV

Changing Bossy Behavior

Inherited traits, such as the tendency to be opinionated and bossy, can be overcome. Here's what it takes:

First, you've got to be convinced that you want to change.

Second, you need to have a plan, such as substituting kind, thoughtful words every time you're tempted to criticize.

Third, make your resolution public. Tell someone, so he or she can support you and encourage you when you feel like giving up, or he or she can remind you when you've failed.

If you fail, don't punish yourself with negative self-talk, such as, "I'm hopeless, why can't I think before I act?" It takes courage and self-worth to change. Negative self-talk destroys that. Instead, apologize and tell yourself, "I can be an understanding parent."

With an "I can" attitude, you can change!

Let all bitterness, wrath, anger, clamor, and evil speaking be put away from you. —Ephesians 4:31, NKJV

DR. KAY KUZMA

Encourage Your Children

Close your eyes and pretend your grown son is flying a kite in an electrical storm. What would you say if you were Ben Franklin's mother? "Can you imagine a man his age out flying a kite in a thunderstorm? He's crazy!" Not many mothers would say, "Keep it up, Ben. You'll be successful yet. There must be some way to harness all that electricity."

How would your child rate you on a scale ranging from highly encouraging to highly discouraging?

It's easy to discourage a child. We do it by being overly critical, by expecting perfection, by being pessimistic, by expressing unrealistic fears, by nagging, and by pointing out weaknesses rather than strengths.

Instead, inspire your child with confidence. With your encouragement, your child can reach his potential and—just like Ben Franklin—be an incredible blessing to others.

"All things are possible to him who believes." —Mark 9:23, NKJV

When the Wrong Answer May Be Right

Educational psychologist Jean Piaget spent a lifetime doing research and writing about cognitive development in children.

One day his daughter was twirling around and became dizzy. "Daddy," she asked, looking up at him, "are things going around for you as they are for me?"

Most of us would consider this the teachable moment to explain the balance mechanism of the inner ear. Instead, he asked, "What do you think?" She shrugged her shoulders, and the teachable moment appeared to be past. But the next day she ran up to her daddy, shouting, "I think I know the answer. Things aren't moving around for you because I'm not tall enough to stir up that much air."

What is more important, the right answer or the thought process?

If Piaget had explained the facts immediately, he would have cut off the thinking involved in his daughter's discovering a solution. Facts are important, but what's really important is that we inspire intellectual curiosity and problem solving in our children.

A wise man will hear and increase learning. —Proverbs 1:5, NKJV

DR. KAY KUZMA

Stop Verbal Abuse

An important family policy is to stick up for the underdog—the person who isn't there at the time to speak up for himself, or isn't assertive enough to set the record straight or stop the verbal abuse.

I remember when we kids would sometimes complain about Mom being unreasonably hard on us, and my dad would always stick up for her. "Children, I won't let you talk about your mom like that. She loves you, and you know you deserved what you got."

We may not have always agreed with Dad's assessment of the situation, but we respected him for sticking up for Mom, and it helped us to be more respectful.

That's what families are for. We all get bent out of shape at times and say things to each other that we shouldn't. But when it happens, someone needs to stand up and set the record straight. "Sorry, kids, I can't allow you to say those hurtful things."

If you want positive family relationships, stop verbal abuse!

"A house divided against a house falls." —Luke 11:17, NKJV

Character Is Caught

What can a parent do to ensure a solid foundation for a child's character development? Here are some essential steps:

1. Show your child you have faith: faith in God, in others, and in your child.
2. Live a virtuous life. Be careful what you watch on TV. Resist the temptation to tell that white lie or to remain silent when the clerk forgets to charge you for something.
3. Continue to seek after knowledge. Let your child see you reading and solving problems.
4. Be temperate. Avoid the afternoon snack or staying up late at night.
5. Be patient even under the most trying circumstances.
6. Respect God and live a godly life.
7. Be a good Samaritan; take time to be thoughtful.
8. Show your children they are loved by spending time together and do loving things for others.

Remember, character is caught—not just taught!

Add to your faith virtue; . . . knowledge; . . . temperance; . . . patience; . . .
godliness; . . . brotherly kindness; and . . . charity. —2 Peter 1:5–7, KJV

DR. KAY KUZMA

Pleasant Time Is Never Wasted Time

James Boswell, the biographer of Samuel Johnson, often talked about the day his father took him fishing and how important it had been to him as a boy. A curious researcher decided to check the father's diary to see whether Boswell's father had recorded a similar reaction to that particular event. And there, opposite the date, these words were penned, "Gone fishing today with my son; a day wasted."

In reality, pleasant time spent with your children is never wasted. It convinces them of your love. Show your wholehearted interest in their affairs, and you'll find your children will blossom with your positive attention. Never let your children think that they're not important to you or that you would rather be doing something else.

Your time given willingly and lovingly is the best gift you can give to your children. It's a gift no money can buy. Give it today, and give it generously.

In Your presence is fullness of joy; at Your right hand are pleasures forevermore. —Psalm 16:11, NKJV

Bitter or Better: It's Your Choice

I've thought a lot about bitterness in connection with my mother's death. What should my response be to the young mother driving a big van who looked back at her children and crossed the center line into my lane, causing a head-on collision and my mother's death?

Should I harbor bitterness? I've decided bitterness and revenge would hurt me more than it would hurt her, and it will never bring Mom back.

When someone wrongs you, it's quite natural to feel anger and bitterness. But these feelings will destroy you if you don't vent them, work through them, forgive the offender, and finally bury the bitterness.

God forgives us. Is it too much to ask that we forgive others? Find a good support group, talk to a professional counselor, and work through those negative feelings. Because of what you've gone through, you can be better, not bitter.

---

*"Forgive, and you will be forgiven." —*Luke 6:37, NKJV

DR. KAY KUZMA

The Expert Authority

There are three types of authority figures. The first is like a policeman or judge, who we fear is going to punish us.

Equally objectionable is the second—the person who imposes his authority over us because of rank, age, or some other type of force. This authority makes us angry.

But the third authority figure is the expert. Parents need to establish this as their type of authority during the first two years of a child's life. This is the person who is so good in his area of expertise that we respect him. We seek his advice and listen carefully when he speaks. It's a great honor to be around this type of authority and a privilege to count a person like this as our friend.

Parents need to be expert authorities to their children. When they are, their children will obey without parents having to force and manipulate.

You slave owners must treat your slaves right, just as I have told them to treat you.
Don't keep threatening them; remember, you yourselves are slaves to Christ;
you have the same Master they do, and he has no favorites. —Ephesians 6:9, TLB

Being Insensitive to Death

Death is a reality of living on this planet, but we must never grow calloused to it. Yet seeing too much death may cause us to grow insensitive.

This became evident to me when, despite our heroic efforts, the puppies from one of our dog's litters just kept dying.

I'm still numb when I think about it! But I didn't cry over the last one that died as I had over the first. And I noticed our children hardly reacted. "Well, another puppy died!" Had seeing too much of death caused them to grow calloused too?

To keep your child sensitive to death, don't just passively accept the deaths shown on TV news stories and in movies. Point out to your child that each person killed was special, each had a grieving family, and each had dreams, desires, and feelings just like the rest of us! And now those are all gone.

Life is precious; don't let familiarity with death take that truth away from your family.

"I have come that they may have life, and that they may have it more abundantly." —John 10:10, NKJV

DR. KAY KUZMA

Be Still and Know Yourself

When was the last time you were completely still and not asleep? How long has it been since your body was at complete rest for maybe an hour or so, and your whole ambition was to listen and think, or just take in the quietness around you?

Today's lifestyle—especially for parents—seems to demand action every single moment of our day. Work, family, social activities, recreation, all contribute to a daily schedule that doesn't allow much time out for anything, especially if that anything is, to all appearances, nothing but stillness.

Lean back or lie down. Close your eyes. What are your innermost thoughts? Have you given your mind time to talk with your heart lately? Time to talk with your Creator?

We all have the time—if we'll just take it. Think of this gift of stillness as a present for yourself.

Rest in the LORD, and wait patiently for Him. —Psalm 37:7, NKJV

The Blessings of Being a Working Mother

Most mothers with jobs have to work to pay the bills. Jobs, however, shouldn't be thought of as something negative. On the contrary, work can be beneficial to the whole family. It all depends on your attitude.

Count the blessings that work brings into your life and the lives of your children: new contacts and friends; new challenges; a focus for your creativity; new ideas to share with your children; colleagues whom your children enjoy; a whole new set of "uncles" and "aunts"; a broadening of interests; and extra income.

Plus, children benefit by seeing their parents willingly taking on different roles; for example, Dad cooking and Mom attending a convention. As children become older, they benefit by feeling needed and by carrying more and more of the home responsibilities. Work can be good for the whole family.

"You shall rejoice in all to which you have put your hand, you and your households, in which the Lord your God has blessed you." —Deuteronomy 12:7, NKJV

DR. KAY KUZMA

Teaching Your Own Children

A father once complained, "Why do I always end up having to help Jason with his homework?" "Be thankful you can help," his wife replied. "Next year you may not know the answers!"

Children grow up so quickly. And it's true; they soon outgrow our limited skills and abilities, moving on to others for special instruction.

Yet, there is a special joy that comes when working side by side with your children, the way Joseph worked with Jesus in the carpenter's shop. And what better method of "training up a child in the way he should go" than by dedicating those first few years to teaching your own children?

I did that with my three until they were almost seven; and although my job didn't allow for homeschooling, I think I would have enjoyed that too. The early years go by so quickly. Take advantage of them. Once they're gone, they're gone!

Train up a child in the way he should go, and when he is old he will not depart from it.
—Proverbs 22:6, NKJV

---

180 POWER TIPS FOR PARENTS

When a Family Member Disappoints You

Holiday times can be tough if you expect a family member to be Prince Charming and he ends up acting more like Bluebeard. Or when you expect Snow White and you get the Wicked Witch.

Uncle Joe promised to be there. He promised he would send a gift. He promised he'd call. And nothing!

Aunt Sue said she would forgive and offer to make restitution. She promised to not be critical. And she ended up making everyone miserable!

What should you do? You can't change them. You've probably been trying for years, and it hasn't worked. And they are members of your family who show up at family gatherings!

The best way to deal with someone who makes life miserable for you is to lower your expectations. Give yourself a chance to grieve over the loss of the idealized family member you wish you had, and accept the family you do have.

If you will do this, what an incredible role model you will be for your kids, especially if some day in the future you unintentionally disappoint them!

God demonstrates His own love toward us, in that while we were still sinners, Christ died for us. —Romans 5:8, NKJV

DR. KAY KUZMA

Running Interference for Your Child

If you have a hyperactive kid, life can be challenging. Not only are you run ragged at home, but chances are you also get criticized when you go out in public, "Why can't you control your child?"

Perhaps the toughest thing, however, is when the rest of the world seems to be down on your child, treating him in harsh, demeaning ways or saying things such as, "Can't you ever do anything right?"

When this happens, you need to take a deep breath and run interference. Don't allow others to degrade your child, especially in public or among his peers. At the same time, you shouldn't make excuses for him so your child feels he can get away with something. Instead, share what you've learned with those who are struggling to find ways to curb his unruly behavior. Teach them a better way by working together with them to find solutions rather than working in opposition.

Don't let people who don't know any better destroy your child's sense of personal value.

Be kind to one another, tenderhearted, forgiving one another,
even as God in Christ forgave you. —Ephesians 4:32, NKJV

Taking Time for Others

My friend told me about a stranger whose visit ran over into family time with their children, which was a very important part of their day. She began to look forward to his departure, not even listening to what he had to say. She was almost ready to tell him that he would need to leave because they had other plans, when she found herself wondering if he were lonely.

"Suddenly," she said, "this visitor was no longer an inconvenience." Instead, it became an opportunity to share a little warmth and friendship that always radiates from a happy family, and they cheerfully invited the stranger to join their family activities.

He willingly participated in their games and even told the kids a great story. Before he left, he thanked them again and again for including him in the evening's fun.

This family didn't have much of the world's riches to give away. They were struggling to make ends meet. But what they had, they gave. And a number of hours later, a much happier man left than the one who had come.

What does your family have to share? Is a little time for the lonely too much to ask of you?

Get into the habit of inviting guests home for dinner or, if they need lodging, for the night. —Romans 12:13, TLB

DR. KAY KUZMA

My Brother's Keeper

Yuck, brothers are bratty. I wish mine were dead." "You ought to have a bossy sister like I have. She drives me up the wall!"

Isn't it sad that so many children grow up thinking it's cool to say hateful things about their brothers or sisters?

A story is told about a girl who needed blood. Her eight-year-old brother had the only type that matched. When asked to give his blood, the boy immediately agreed. During the procedure both children were lying side by side, and then at the end, the little girl was wheeled out of the room first.

The physician then looked over at the boy and saw tears in his eyes. When he went to comfort him, the boy asked, "When am I going to die?"

The physician explained he wasn't going to die, and then asked, "Because you thought that by giving your blood you were going to die, why did you do it?"

The boy answered, "Well, she is my sister, and I love her."

If only more kids felt this way about their brothers and sisters!

"Am I my brother's keeper?" —Genesis 4:9, NKJV

Fill Your Emotional Container With Joy

Think of yourself as an emotional container. There is only so much room inside you for feelings. When you are filled with negative feelings, it's difficult to experience anything positive.

One way to get rid of those troublesome negative feelings is to write them down. The process of dealing with the feeling takes it out of your emotional container, creating a void inside you.

Now you have two choices: either continue thinking about that negative feeling you wrote down so it has a chance to jump back inside, or fill the void with something positive.

Start the filling process by thinking of something for which you are thankful. As long as your mind dwells on something positive, it can't concentrate on the negative.

If you continue this exercise until all the negatives have been changed to positives, your cup will overflow with joy.

In Your presence is fullness of joy; at Your right hand are pleasures forevermore. —Psalm 16:11, NKJV

DR. KAY KUZMA

The String Strategy

You're not going to be able to control all your children's squabbles, but you can get rid of the conflicts between you and your children by remembering that children are very much like strings.

Children want to win; they want to be in control. Rather than fighting over the issue, it is better to avoid as much conflict as possible. A string will help you to remember what to do.

If you stretch a string out straight and push one end of the string in the direction you want it to go, it will buckle under the pressure of being pushed. Children, when pushed, forced, and manipulated, will tend to resist. Instead, take the other end of the string and lead the string in the direction you want it to go, and it will follow.

Children will too. If you learn to motivate, encourage, influence, and lead them in the right direction, rather than forcing them, everyone wins!

The Lord is my shepherd. . . . He leads me beside the still waters. He restores my soul;
He leads me in the paths of righteousness for His name's sake. —Psalm 23:1–3, NKJV

Ten Parenting Dos and Don'ts

Here is a list that's going to help you be a better parent, so take note. The list is based on a worldwide survey of one hundred thousand children, asking what things they wanted their parents to do or not do. Here is their top ten:

1. Treat all your children with equal affection.
2. Keep close to them.
3. Make their friends welcome in your home.
4. Don't quarrel in front of them.
5. Be thoughtful of each other.
6. Never lie to your children.
7. Always answer their questions.
8. Don't punish them in the presence of others.
9. Be consistent in affection and moods.
10. Concentrate on good points, not on failings.

Well, there you have it, the ten most important things kids want from parents. How do you measure up?

Woe to those who are wise in their own eyes, and prudent in their own sight! —Isaiah 5:21, NKJV

DR. KAY KUZMA

A Safe-Place Policy

Just how safe are your kids at home? Not from dangerous tools, fire, and things like that, but from those words and actions that can hurt just as badly.

A mother once wrote to me saying, "We were discouraged when we moved to this neighborhood six years ago because the children were so cruel to one another. So I implemented a 'safe-place policy.' No one playing here in our home or yard would be teased by another, hurt by another, or made fun of."

She ended her letter with this story: "Late one afternoon there was a lot of commotion on our porch. I opened the door in time to hear the child who was standing there shouting to the bully in the street, 'Go on home and leave us alone. You can't bother us here, 'cuz we're in the holy yard.' "

I love the idea. Think how different life would be for children if every home had a "safe-place policy" and a "holy yard"!

Whoever trusts in the LORD shall be safe. —Proverbs 29:25, NKJV

Motivation for a Savings Account

Have you ever wished for that pot of gold at the end of the rainbow? There are times we all need extra money. That's why I'm glad my husband set up a savings account for us when we were first married. You know, we never missed those extra dollars that went into the account each month, but they sure came in handy when we needed them.

You can motivate your children to start a savings account if you let them know that at their high-school graduation, you'll match whatever amount they have saved. Or if they want a car, you will match whatever they have saved toward it.

Make it possible for your children to earn money so they can measure their expensive tastes by how many hours of work it took them to accumulate that amount of money. When viewed from that perspective, expensive tastes become much more practical, and your kids will find it easier to save.

To win the contest you must deny yourselves many things that would keep you from doing your best.
—1 Corinthians 9:25, TLB

DR. KAY KUZMA

Play the What-If Game

When life is a rat race, the routine boring, and you don't have time for your kids, play the what-if game to discover some alternatives. For example, what would happen if you quit work or worked only part time or said, "No overtime"? What would happen if you went back to school or decided to change jobs or to move?

To play the game fairly, you must remain open to a wide range of possible answers to each question you pose.

That's exactly what Bruce Schneider did. He was an aeronautics engineer; his wife, an artist. They played the what-if game, downsized, left big-city jobs, and moved to the country with their children. Bruce applied his engineering expertise to sculpturing—which was something he could do at home.

His success exceeded his wildest expectations. But the real benefit was more time with his wife and children and no more guilt. If families like the Schneiders can do this, you can too. And it all starts with the question, "What if . . . ?"

"If you have faith as a mustard seed, you will say to this mountain, 'Move . . .' and nothing will be impossible."
—Matthew 17:20, NKJV

Guilt Drives Parents to Make Mistakes

Do you feel guilty you're not spending enough time with your kids? If so, be careful. Guilt can lead you to make six big mistakes.

Mistake 1 is overprotecting your child by not allowing your child out of your sight when you are there. Children thrive on age-related independence—not on smothering.

Mistake 2 is giving unnecessary gifts. But presents never take the place of parental presence.

Giving in to demands is mistake 3. Children often play on a parent's guilt feelings to get what they want.

Mistake 4 is feeling sorry for your children. But this only encourages them to feel sorry for themselves.

To avoid mistake 5, don't allow your children to escape home responsibilities by doing things for them that they should be doing for themselves.

And to avoid mistake 6, don't ignore misbehavior.

Instead of allowing guilt to control you, control it by choosing to spend meaningful time with your kids.

Do not withhold correction from a child. —Proverbs 23:13, NKJV

DR. KAY KUZMA

Labels That Stick

Have you ever accidently superglued your finger to an object? Ouch! It's almost impossible to get it off without tearing away your skin.

Negative labels stick like superglue. "John's crazy." "What a klutz." "She's a loser." "Dave's just a big baby." "Joe's a cheat." Say these things to a kid once, and it's likely to stick forever. Even though children try to forget, the negative labels keep popping up in their minds. Before long, kids begin to believe these things are really true.

Positive labels take longer to stick. Labels such as, "What a great worker! You're thoughtful," are more like regular glue.

The moral is to apply positive labels liberally and often. But when it comes to negative labels, watch out. Criticism, faultfinding, and negative labeling have superglue properties that stick immediately—and too often, permanently.

Some people like to make cutting remarks, but the words of the wise soothe and heal. —Proverbs 12:18, TLB

Take the Kids Along

Have you ever thought of taking the kids along on a business trip? Too expensive? Not necessarily! There are ways you can cut the costs. Try last-minute airline tickets, newspaper or online specials, or get reservations far enough ahead to get economy rates.

Shop around for competitive hotels that will let the family stay for one rate. Unlimited mileage on car rentals allows the family to sightsee while you are in meetings. And if you don't mind fixing some of your own meals or taking advantage of fast-food places rather than the hotel restaurant, you can save considerably.

But regardless of the cost, the benefits of taking your family along on a business trip can outweigh the expense. When Kevin was twelve, I took him on a trip to Florida with me. After my speaking appointment, we spent two extra days at the Epcot Center. What great memories!

Children can gain so much from being with their parents and seeing new places. Also, it's a great way to let the family know that they are an important priority in your life. So why not consider taking the family along on your next trip?

I conclude that, first, there is nothing better for a man than to be happy and to enjoy himself as long as he can;
and second, that he should eat and drink and enjoy the fruits of his labors,
for these are gifts from God. —Ecclesiastes 3:12, 13, TLB

DR. KAY KUZMA

A Tribute to Parents

I enjoy asking people I admire, "What did your parents do right?" One unforgettable story was about O. D. and Ruth McKee, founders of McKee Foods, well known for their Little Debbie snack products!

The McKee kids remember helping their dad plant a half-acre field of tomatoes. Dad led the family assembly line with a cut-off broom handle to poke deep holes in the soft soil, followed by child 1 dropping a tomato plant beside each hole, child 2 placing the plant in position in the hole, child 3 watering, and child 4 firmly tapping the soil in place.

Even though both Mom and Dad put in long hours at the fast-growing bakery they owned and could have hired workers to plant those tomatoes, they did not let the training of their children suffer. In the McKee family, everyone learned to work—and they worked as a team.

I think we can learn something from successful families, don't you?

Work brings profit; talk brings poverty! —Proverbs 14:23, TLB

What My Dad Gave Me

My dad gave me three gifts that can never be taken away. They didn't cost him any money. But today, they're the most priceless treasures I possess. The first: Dad gave me the feeling of being special. The second gift: he loved my mom. And three: he gave me the gift of optimism!

Three simple gifts, but they have made me what I am today.

What did your dad give you? You may not have very positive feelings about your dad. Maybe he abandoned the family or abused you when he got drunk. Dads have made a lot of mistakes. But don't let those mistakes fill you with bitterness and take away your joy of living.

Forgive your dad and begin thinking of the special things he gave you. Maybe it was the twinkle in his eye, his laugh, or the way he valued freedom. Every dad gives something positive to his kids. Look for it, hold on to it, and say Thank you!

Now consider, What gifts are you giving to your children?

Only a fool despises his father's advice; a wise son considers each suggestion. —Proverbs 15:5, TLB

DR. KAY KUZMA

Make a Why-Not List

Kids love surprises. They like to try new things and have a change in routine. And what better time than now to break out of your rut and say, "Why not?"

Why not have a hot dog and marshmallow roast in your backyard? Or better yet, pitch a tent and have a backyard campout. We did this a few times when we were kids—and loved it! We had the fun of sleeping on air mattresses and in sleeping bags, while our parents could enjoy their comfortable bed inside. And we all had the convenience of indoor plumbing when nature called!

Kids love water fights. Find some squirt bottles and get the whole family involved! Or try a three-legged race!

Start a wildflower, insect, or rock collection. Go bird-watching at dawn. Visit the local dairy, sugar-beet refinery, baking plant, or whatever industry you have in your local area. Float boats on the pond in the park or feed the ducks.

It's time to abandon your routine, say, "Why not?" and make a meaningful memory for your family.

It is senseless for you to work so hard from early morning until late at night. —Psalm 127:2, TLB

The Most Creative Job in the World

There was a full one-page ad that appeared in the *Wall Street Journal* a number of years ago that I'll never forget. In big bold print it read, "The Most Creative Job in the World." And then it continued, "It involves taste, fashion, decorating, recreation, education, transportation, psychology, romance, cuisine, designing, literature, medicine, handicraft, art, horticulture, economics, government, community relations, pediatrics, geriatrics, entertainment, maintenance, purchasing, direct mail, law, accounting, religion, energy and management."

The final punch line was, "Anyone who can handle all those has to be somebody special. She is. She's a homemaker."

If you sometimes feel discouraged as a parent, remember you have the most creative job in the world—and by far, the most important.

Praise her for the many fine things she does. These good deeds of hers shall bring her honor and recognition from even the leaders of the nations. —Proverbs 31:31, TLB

DR. KAY KUZMA

Tough Times Are Great for Families

It's not necessarily the good times that draw a family closer; it's struggling to overcome the bad ones. It's meeting difficulties and, together, surviving them, such as on a camping trip when the tent blows down in the middle of the night or the car breaks down a hundred miles from nowhere. These will be the times that you will recount at family reunions over the years.

Gary Smalley, a counselor and author, has said that when he was a young father, he noticed that there was one common factor in strong, healthy families. They all went camping. So he determined his family was going to spend time camping. Now after years of experiences, he realizes it wasn't the camping that brings families together. It's the problems they overcame while camping.

So face each problem with courage and a smile, knowing that it's just another pillar that's going to make your family strong.

Is your life full of difficulties and temptations? Then be happy, for when the way is rough,
your patience has a chance to grow. —James 1:2, 3, TLB

What Have We Done to Our Kids?

Violence has become a common part of life in our society: child abuse, family violence, gangs, war. But I was stunned as I read about a study on one college campus: "As many as one dating couple out of five, regularly beats each other up and accepts pushes, punches, slaps and kicks, as the tax on romance."

I have always been opposed to violence. But to realize that love has become so perverted that couples think they have to accept abuse as a part of a love relationship is indeed sad.

The article ended with this interesting observation, "Was it Oscar Wilde who observed that 'we always hurt the one we love?' . . . And was it you and I, just yesterday, who assured kids, while we were punishing them, that 'I'm doing this because I love you'?"

What have we done to our kids? It's something to think about, isn't it!

Your own soul is nourished when you are kind; it is destroyed when you are cruel.
—Proverbs 11:17, TLB

DR. KAY KUZMA

Just a Phone Call Away

Children feel more secure when they know that their working mom is just a phone call away. A number of years ago at certain businesses, it was impossible to make a business call between three and four o'clock in the afternoon because the lines were clogged with kids calling their moms.

"Mommy, Shawnee won't clean the living room!"

Five minutes later, it was Shawnee. "Mommy, Jonathan is bugging me."

A few minutes later, "Mommy, may I make some macaroni?" Or, "We can't get the cat out of the tree." Or, "Mom, thanks for those guppies you got me." Ten minutes later, "Mom, how can you tell if a guppy's pregnant?"

We may not have to worry about clogged business lines now that most moms carry cell phones, but have you noticed how many of those cell phones ring right about the time the kids get home from school—and ring again and again?

It's great to be just a phone call—or a text message—away, but don't let your kids abuse this privilege.

A person with good sense is respected. —Proverbs 13:15, NLT

What Kids Think of Marriage

What exactly is marriage? Well, just ask a child—and you're bound to get some very interesting answers. For example, Eric, age six, said, "Marriage is when you get to keep your girl and don't have to give her back to her parents!"

Eight-year-old Carolyn said the proper age to get married is "eighty-four! Because at that age, you don't have to work anymore, and you can spend all your time loving each other in your bedroom."

And as far as deciding whom to marry? Carolyn comments, "My mother says to look for a man who is kind. That's what I'll do. . . . I'll find somebody who's kinda tall and handsome."

You might laugh at what these children say. But what your children are learning about marriage from you is no laughing matter. Do they see marriage as a love-filled relationship where you enjoy meeting each other's needs? Ideally, they do. Because it's quite likely they'll pattern their marriages after yours!

May the Lord continually bless you with heaven's blessings as well as with human joys. —Psalm 128:5, TLB

DR. KAY KUZMA

Love and Limits—the Answer to Rebellion

How do you handle a rebellious kid? The best prescription is love and limits—in big doses! Children are like icebergs. The tip—the rebellious behavior that is noticeable—is not the entire iceberg. The biggest part of an iceberg is under the surface of the water. It's the same way with children who are acting out. The biggest problem is not the rebellious behavior; it's what lies underneath the surface—the negative emotions causing the rebellion.

When the negative emotions are dealt with and defused, the rebellious behavior will melt away. The problem is, how do you get to those negative emotions? That's where love and limits fit in. You must give your child enough love to crowd out and replace those negative emotions, while, at the same time, you must hold tightly to enough limits so the child's rebellious behavior doesn't hurt the child, others, or things.

And if you need professional guidance on how to do this, get it! Don't let things get worse.

Knowing what is right to do and then not doing it is sin. —James 4:17, TLB

Helping Children Deal With Death

It's not always possible to shield children from death. One moment a family may be laughing and singing as they drive along the highway and the next—the sickening crunch of metal, and the life of a family member or friend has been snuffed out. And for children, the death of a loved pet can be a terrible blow.

Because we can't escape this reality, it's important for us to know how to help children through the grieving process.

Make sure your children don't feel irrational guilt, that they were somehow to blame.

Don't exclude children from family gatherings or memorial services; but don't force them to participate either!

Allow your children to work through fears and fantasies about death in their play. For example, if they want to have a funeral for a dead pet, let them.

You can't shield your children from death, but you can offer them a compassionate heart, a listening ear, and the hope of resurrection when Jesus comes again.

"Blessed are those who mourn, for they shall be comforted." —Matthew 5:4, NKJV

DR. KAY KUZMA

Reward the Positive

You can learn a lot about children by raising a puppy. Puppies are so eager to please. They will learn to do all sorts of unnatural things, like playing dead, singing, or shaking hands, all because they know they will be rewarded.

It's the same with children. They have an inner desire to please and will try hard to be good if they know it brings a reward such as a smile or a compliment. But without thinking, we often give more attention to our children's wrong actions than we give for what is right—and we reinforce their misbehavior!

So, begin noticing the positive things children do. Let them overhear you telling someone else something nice about them. Comment on the creative projects they make. And give them plenty of nonverbal positive strokes, such as a hug, a wink, or a smile.

Children, like puppies, will do anything for a little attention, so make sure you give it when they're good.

"Rejoice and be exceedingly glad, for great is your reward in heaven." —Matthew 5:12, NKJV

Eye Contact and Bonding

Eye contact is critical for the development of healthy relationships! Watch new parents. Without coaching, most will immediately position their newborns in their arms in such a way that they can look at their baby's eyes. And isn't it interesting that the baby focuses best at about eight inches—just the distance that is normally between the eyes of babies when they are held and their parents' eyes?

Eye contact continues to be important for bonding throughout life. What is one of the clearest ways to distinguish two lovers in a crowd from just ordinary friends? Isn't it the way they gaze at each other?

And when you want to tell your children something important, if you get down at their level and look them in the eye, they will listen more carefully and remember better.

How much time do you spend looking at the significant people in your life? Do you take time for some eye-to-eye contact each day? I hope so, because eye contact is great relational bonding material!

Look upon me and be merciful to me, as Your custom is toward those who love Your name.
—Psalm 119:132, NKJV

DR. KAY KUZMA

Getting Kids Hooked on Reading

Reading is a window to the world. If your children don't open that window naturally, you need to make reading as meaningful and attractive as possible.

Start by spending thirty minutes a day reading to them. You think you don't have the time? You can find it. Read to them while they do the dishes, fold the clothes, or clean their rooms. If you can't coordinate your schedules, read aloud to yourself and record the chapter so your kids can listen later.

After getting your children hooked on a good book, buy them the next book of a series, and read the first chapter to them. I wouldn't be surprised if they pick it up and finish reading it themselves.

You'll find children do more reading if you turn off the TV, take away the video games, and provide a pleasant reading nook where they can snuggle into comfortable chairs. And remember, example speaks louder than words! So pick up a good book yourself and throw open that "window to the world."

You are our epistle written in our hearts, known and read by all men. —2 Corinthians 3:2, NKJV

Get to Know Your Kids' Friends and Families

Parents, you have a responsibility to know who your children are hanging out with. It would be easy if you could go by looks. But there could be some great kids dressed up in black leather jackets, tight torn jeans, and purple hair. So, you must make a real effort to get to know these kids. Make your home an attractive gathering place for the neighborhood kids. Feed them and listen.

Next, get to know their parents. Have a neighborhood party. Invite each family over for dessert. Plan a time when the parents can talk together when the kids aren't around. Discuss parenting issues such as drugs, alcohol, premarital sex, violence, and gangs. Talk about the values that you feel are important and how you can work together to make sure the kids are making healthy lifestyle choices. Exchange phone numbers.

Let your children know that you, as their parents, are cooperating in supervising their activities. For the safety and health of your kids, stay involved!

There are "friends" who pretend to be friends, but there is a friend who sticks closer than a brother.
—Proverbs 18:24, TLB

DR. KAY KUZMA

Give Your Child a Gold Medal for Efficiency

Motivation is the key to efficiency. Remember the efficiency-expert father in that classic film *Cheaper by the Dozen*? Remember how he was always timing his kids?

If you want efficiency, maybe it's time to get out your stopwatch and offer a gold medal each time a child achieves a personal record! Give him a quarter for a job completed in a certain amount of time. If it takes longer, decrease the reward.

On a bulletin board, post official family records for doing various chores, and encourage the children to beat their own records.

Hold a contest among family members to see who can devise ways to do routine tasks more quickly. For example, see if the table can be cleared in one trip if everyone carries as much as possible in a "two-hand takeoff."

And ban TV until after work is done. It's amazing how much motivation can be generated when your children's favorite program airs in fifteen minutes!

Inspiring kids to do jobs around the house is important, but teaching them to do those tasks efficiently is just as important.

Let all things be done decently and in order. —1 Corinthians 14:40, NKJV

Listen Before Punishing

Dad's rule was, "No yelling when I'm on the phone." One evening his young son ran to him screaming. Dad hung up the phone, and when his son wouldn't quit screaming, he spoke harshly to him and finally spanked him for disturbing his call.

Later, Dad learned the reason for the screaming. His son had fallen and hurt his back. If only Dad had listened before punishing!

Much of the negative behavior seen in children, such as running away, threatening suicide, or yelling words of hate, is merely the child's crude way of saying, "Mom, Dad, please listen to me!"

Let's face it, most of us don't take time to listen carefully to the messages our children are trying to send. And, consequently, we aren't as understanding as we should be. We end up saying what's on our minds and hurting our children in the process—cutting off their attempts to communicate. Remember what it says in Proverbs 1:5 (NKJV), "A wise man will hear and increase learning."

You must all be quick to listen, slow to speak, and slow to get angry. —James 1:19, NLT

DR. KAY KUZMA

Why Kids Hate Cleaning Their Rooms

Why don't children like to clean their rooms? Turn that question around. Think of things your children really like to do and ask them why.

Their answers may vary, but probably because it was fun. Friends are doing it. Their friends value this activity. They want to impress their friends. Others appreciate what they're doing. Others notice. It enhances a skill that is important to them. It helps them toward a goal they want to accomplish. They get rewards that are meaningful to them. It's easy and doesn't seem like work. It makes them and others happy. It makes them feel competent. They take personal ownership and have an investment in the outcome. And the list could go on.

Now to solve the problem of kids not liking to clean their rooms, all you have to do is build the above elements into the task, and you should end up with children who love to clean their rooms! Good luck!

An empty stable stays clean—but there is no income from an empty stable. —Proverbs 14:4, TLB

A Riddle of Love

Do you enjoy riddles? Remember the one about what's black and white and read all over? The answer: a newspaper. Here's another riddle that isn't as well known, but should be because it is the key to raising happy, well-adjusted children. *What's the only thing you can give away and end up with more?*

The answer: love. That's right. If you fill up another person so full of love that they can't seem to contain it, the chances are great that something nice will come back to you.

Love is an abstract concept, but it becomes more concrete when you think of people as having love cups that either empty or fill, depending upon what happens to them. The substance that fills a love cup is attention—positive attention. The more you give, the more you get. Teach this riddle to your children, and encourage them to be love-cup fillers.

Dear friends, let us practice loving each other, for love comes from God and those who are loving and kind show that they are the children of God, and that they are getting to know him better. —1 John 4:7, TLB

DR. KAY KUZMA

Teaching Children Responsibility

Don't become angry and frustrated at your children's lack of responsibility. Anger doesn't help! Instead, it will only make them feel bad about themselves and will lower their respect for you as an authority figure.

Instead, to increase their motivation, make a game out of the tasks you want them to accomplish. Then reward them for small pieces of the task as soon as they are done, instead of waiting until the entire project is complete. Children thrive on immediate gratification.

If you expect your children to be responsible for cleaning their rooms, simplify the task by putting out of reach the things they don't need regularly. Too many things become distracting, and at the end of the day their rooms will be colossal messes that are too big for them to handle without major protests and floods of tears.

Then pray for patience and kind understanding.

Love is very patient and kind. —1 Corinthians 13:4, TLB

Polite Children Are Trained Children

How do you teach children to be polite and to say "Please," "Thank you," "You're welcome," "Excuse me," and all those other nice comments that show others respect?

You've heard the saying, "You can't teach old dogs new tricks." Well, it's not impossible to teach older children to be polite, but it's certainly more difficult. The older your children get before they see polite behavior modeled by others and are required themselves to act politely, the more difficult it will be to teach them.

Start by modeling the polite behavior you expect. Tell your child how to respond, and then reward him or her immediately with a smile, a wink, or some other acknowledgement of praise. The training of polite behavior is achieved by a stimulus-response-reward pattern that is, believe it or not, used successfully when training animals. Just remember, the key to successful training is consistency.

"Inasmuch as you did it to one of the least of these My brethren, you did it to Me." —Matthew 25:40, NKJV

DR. KAY KUZMA

Nice Parents

Trying to be nice can get parents into trouble, if *nice* means you smile at wrongdoing and fail to impose meaningful consequences that would teach your children valuable lessons about right and wrong.

"No gain without pain," is a common saying, and it certainly applies to moral development. Lessons that help a child (or adult) become a better person are often painful. And yet these very lessons may build a child's sense of personal value. How?

First, children sense they are valuable when people are willing to take their time to teach them to become better persons.

Second, improved behavior brought about by discipline means that others will react more positively to your children and may even spend more time with them, making them feel even more important.

Third, when children know they are doing what they should be doing, their self-respect is increased.

Be a nice parent and teach your children to be nice kids!

Obey your spiritual leaders and be willing to do what they say. —Hebrews 13:17, TLB

Help Kids Feel Desirable and Competent

If you want to preserve and build your child's sense of personal value, you must discipline in such a way as to make your child feel desirable and competent.

Young children who are not able to take care of all their own personal needs often feel incompetent. That's why self-worth in childhood is primarily determined by how desirable they feel. And that's why children so often fall victim to feelings of inferiority.

Parents who complain about, argue with, ignore, or criticize a child when the reason for the child's "misbehavior" is unmet needs, can destroy the child's feelings of desirability. Their message is "I don't like you," or "I don't want to be around you."

To preserve your child's personal value, correct, but do it in such a way that your child still feels desirable and competent.

"Be merciful, just as your Father also is merciful." —Luke 6:36, NKJV

DR. KAY KUZMA

Underage Policemen Aren't Appreciated

Do you have an underage "policeman" in your home? One who lets you know every possible misstep of the other sisters and brothers? "Mommy, Todd is teasing the girls, and Lisa is using your perfume."

It gets on your nerves, doesn't it? You want your children to develop clear standards of what is right and wrong, but you also want them to develop a certain sense of sibling loyalty. No one likes a tattletale!

You can stop this tattling behavior in your home by ignoring it. When your junior policeman comes to you with a hot tidbit, say in a cool, disinterested voice, "Oh," or, "Too bad," and go about your work. Children tattle because of what's in it for them, perhaps to get a closer relationship with Mom or to get back at sister. Don't fall into their trap. Break this negative habit now, and turn that junior policeman back into a child and a loyal sibling.

Where there is no wood, the fire goes out; and where there is no talebearer, strife ceases.
—Proverbs 26:20, NKJV

Why Children Ask "Why?"

Have you ever wondered why children always ask "Why"?
Children have an innate curiosity to understand their world. "Why?" starts out as a method to get more information. However, because children's questions often come at a time when parents are in a hurry, their curt response tends to stir up more questions.

Take those questions seriously. Immediately give your children the information and the attention they desire, and you'll find the why questions will be asked more and more to get information, rather than as an indirect way of trying to get attention.

The next time your child asks, "Why?" stop what you are doing, bend down to her level, look her in the eyes, and give a short, simple answer. Then ask, "Do you understand?" Chances are she will, and her curiosity will be satisfied!

Whatever you do, do it with kindness and love. —1 Corinthians 16:14, TLB

DR. KAY KUZMA

Self-Help for Depression

Have you ever felt like saying, "I'm going to go eat worms!" When you feel that way, worms aren't going to help. But you can do something that will!

- Take time to contact a family member or friend who makes you feel warm inside. If no one comes to mind, you may need to enlarge your circle of friends.
- Force yourself to reach out and do something nice for someone.
- Read or listen to something uplifting. Search for Bible promises or listen to uplifting music.
- Get some exercise. A long walk in the fresh air will do wonders.
- Put your house or apartment in order. A messy place can be depressing.
- Start planning something that you've always wanted to do. Write down your dream and develop a plan of action that will lead to fulfillment. Then make yourself get up and start on step one.

Delight yourself also in the LORD, and He shall give you the desires of your heart. —Psalm 37:4, NKJV

Listening to Feelings

A frustrated wife wrote, "My husband is always telling me what to do, when all I want him to do is listen and try to understand me!"

I answered, "He may be uncomfortable with the expression of feelings. When something is wrong, the immediate tendency for most men is to fix it. But you can't hold on to feelings and fix them as you would the battery of a car. Yet your husband probably doesn't realize this, and therefore he tries to fix your feelings by telling you what to do."

It takes practice to be a good listener. I suggest you start when you have no major emotional issues facing the two of you. Look in each other's eyes and let each talk for two minutes without interruption, with the other occasionally saying, "Oh," "Yes," "That's interesting," or some other expression that says, "I'm listening." Then give the other a turn. Practice makes perfect!

Walk in love, as Christ also has loved us and given Himself for us. —Ephesians 5:2, NKJV

DR. KAY KUZMA

Presence Versus Presents

Things never truly satisfy. Relationships do! But for many it's easier to give some object or thing than to give oneself, because to give oneself takes one's valuable time. So, after an exhausting day at work, many parents feel it's easier to bring home some trinket to an attention-starved child than to spend time together.

I believe fewer things would be purchased for children if parents really evaluated their motives for giving.

Great reasons for giving are if the child needs it, or if the gift would contribute to the child's learning and enhance the child's potential in some way. Another valid reason would be that the gift contributes to family togetherness or a sense of team spirit.

Just because you feel guilty or because your children want something doesn't mean they should have it. Instead, try giving some of your time. It's the best present of all!

"If you then, being evil, know how to give good gifts to your children, how much more will your Father who is in heaven give good things to those who ask Him!" —Matthew 7:11, NKJV

Word Pictures Speak Louder Than Words

Alice was having trouble getting her kids to understand how she felt when she would ask them to do something and they totally ignored her. She tried to share her feelings in words, but they seemed to fall on deaf ears.

She finally got her point across when she told them a story. "Once upon a time, there was a mother who loved her children very much. She took good care of them, fed them delicious meals, washed their clothes, and willingly chauffeured them to their many activities. Then one day, as they were walking through a forest, the mother stepped into some quicksand and began to sink. She yelled for her children to help her, but they totally ignored her calls until she sank out of sight and died." Mom then ended her word picture with, "That's how I feel every time I ask you for help." The kids got the message, apologized, and the next time she made a request, they all jumped up to help.

I've heard it said that a picture is worth a thousand words. Paint a word picture for your kids, and see if it doesn't help them get the message.

Be kind to one another, tenderhearted, forgiving one another,
just as God in Christ also forgave you. —Ephesians 4:32, NKJV

DR. KAY KUZMA

How to Manage a Zoo and Monkeys Too

Is your life sometimes so hectic you feel like you're running a zoo? If so, you need to picture all those things that you think you have to do as monkeys—a bunch of jabbering, demanding monkeys clinging on your back, pulling your hair, and poking fingers in your eyes.

How long would you put up with real monkeys in your life? Probably not five minutes. You would get rid of them!

You've got to do the same with all those things that you "think" need to be done, but don't really contribute to your family. Think of them as monkeys. You can manage only so many without losing control. Separate those monkeys (things that are vying for your attention) into two groups: Those you really love, and those that you merely tolerate. Then, either give the unwanted ones away or let them die.

Cruel? It's the only way to manage the zoo and be a good parent too!

To everything there is a season. . . . A time to gain, and a time to lose; a time to keep, and a time to throw away. —Ecclesiastes 3:1, 6, NKJV

Persistence

I'm a sanguine, so it's easy for me to blame my temperament style for some of my faults. One of the worst, I think, is the scatterbrain way I work on projects. I go to my computer to write a radio script and see the plant on my desk needs watering. I get up to water it and notice some crumbs on the floor. Then I remember we need a loaf of bread, so I write it on the shopping list. The phone rings. It's about my next speaking trip, and I run for my appointment book and—two days later I remember, oh yes, the radio script!

I'm working on this problem, and here's a jingle I found helpful:

> *One thing at a time and that done well,*
> *Is a very good thing as all may tell.*
> *Work with your will and all your might.*
> *Things done by halves are never done right!*

Do you or one of your children have trouble focusing on a task until it's done? If so, hopefully this jingle will help you too.

One thing I do, forgetting those things which are behind and reaching forward to those things which are ahead,
I press toward the goal for the prize of the upward call of God in Christ Jesus.
—Philippians 3:13, 14, NKJV

DR. KAY KUZMA

Breakfast With Your Family

I used to think it was hard getting the family together when they were just preschoolers, but when the kids were teenagers it was worse. With school and work schedules, eating lunch together was impossible, and supper was almost as bad. That's why I made it a rule in our house that breakfast was family time. At least we could start the day together.

But, above and beyond the importance of time together, research indicates that eating breakfast is good for your health and aids in academic achievement. When breakfast is skipped, children show decreased problem-solving ability, lower test scores, and increased error rates.

So, get up fifteen minutes earlier tomorrow morning. Fix one simple dish. Try peanut-buttered toast topped with hot applesauce and sliced bananas and blueberries, and treat your family to the best possible start for a great day—by starting it together.

Jesus said to them, "Come and eat breakfast." —John 21:12, NKJV

Four Foundations of Parenting

For more than forty years, I have sorted and sifted through hundreds of child-rearing concepts to discover the essential building stones to a healthy, happy, spiritually sensitive individual. I've discovered four.

The first is LOVE. That feeling that my parents will accept me regardless of what I do.

DISCIPLINE is next because without limits and consequences, it's almost impossible to become self-disciplined. But you can safely discipline only as much as you are willing to love.

Developing CHARACTER must not be ignored. Children must know how to make good moral decisions and avoid negative peer pressure.

And the fourth cornerstone? SELF-WORTH. Unless children feel good about who they are, they will never have the confidence necessary to become everything God gifted them to become.

Unless the Lord builds the house, they labor in vain who build it. —Psalm 127:1, NKJV

DR. KAY KUZMA

Stop, Look, and Listen

S top, look, and listen. I bet your mom or dad gave you those instructions when you were small when you had to cross a busy street or the railroad tracks. Mine did!

But stop, look, and listen is also great advice to parents who want their children to continue to share with them what's on their hearts.

Children crave positive attention from their parents and other significant persons in their lives. It makes them feel loved when you show an interest in their activities. It also gives you valuable subject matter for engaging in meaningful conversations with them in the future.

So when your children say something, pay attention. Stop what you're doing. Look at them. Listen to what they say. Make appropriate comments. Watch your children's body language for clues to hidden messages, and be willing to clarify what they are trying to say rather than jumping to conclusions and leaving both you and your children frustrated!

Answer me speedily, O LORD; my spirit fails! Do not hide Your face from me,
lest I be like those who go down into the pit. —Psalm 143:7, NKJV

Salvaging Red-Traffic-Light Time

I remember that when we first moved to Redlands, California, I could drive to my work at Loma Linda University in twelve minutes. Down San Bernardino Avenue to the freeway and off at Anderson. Twenty years later, and a million more cars, it took twenty-four minutes. No, we hadn't moved. But traffic lights had gone up on almost every corner! What a waste of time sitting there waiting for a green light!

Not long ago I read that the average motorist spends twenty-six hours a year waiting for traffic signals to change. I know I've spent at least that much. And then I got to thinking. What if, instead of getting upset at the delay, I would use that red-light time to memorize inspirational thoughts, plan something fun to do with the children, or pray for someone?

Think about what you would like to accomplish if given twenty-six more hours a year, and begin to use your red-light time productively.

There is a time for everything, and a season for every activity under heaven. —Ecclesiastes 3:1, NIV

DR. KAY KUZMA

Walking the Parental Tightrope

If you had a choice about whether you would walk a plank or a tightrope across a raging river, which would you choose? The plank, of course. There is a much broader margin for error.

Parenting is much the same. The greater our loving commitment to our children, as shown by the time spent together, the broader the plank we walk. We might make some mistakes, perhaps lean too far one way or the other, but we have room to make a correction. Within the space of the time spent together, we can still get the message of love across to our children.

The less time spent together, however, the narrower the plank. When you're down to a tightrope, watch out. You can't afford to make any mistakes, become angry, or criticize. On a tightrope, the least amount of negative friction between parent and child can destroy your relationship.

May the Lord continually bless you with heaven's blessings as well as with human joys. —Psalm 128:5, TLB

Can Grouchy Attitudes Be Dangerous?

Sometimes older folks can be grouchy and bitter, especially if they are going through hard times or illness. Does that mean you shouldn't let your children spend time with them since kids are so easily influenced? No, children need to learn how to be kind to people of all ages without picking up their bad habits. In addition, kids can have a softening effect on unhappy people.

If your children begin picking up embittered attitudes or the sarcastic words of older folks, you will need to make it clear that you can't allow your kids to act that way.

Sometimes an adult's sharp words hurt children's feelings. When this happens, explain to your kids, "Some older people don't know any better. It's our job to accept people just the way they are, *but we don't have to be like them.*" Then allow your children to honestly say to the offender, "Your words hurt my feelings," or "You're emptying my love cup." Children might not be able to change an elderly person's behavior—but they don't need to copy it!

Let all bitterness, wrath, anger, clamor, and evil speaking be put away from you. —Ephesians 4:31, NKJV

DR. KAY KUZMA

How Important Is Family?

Every family is made up of different personalities, not all of whom are easy to get along with. Members of extended families who are able to retain close relationships are those who respect each other and feel good enough about themselves that they hold no grudges against the others.

A relationship takes two people. And in some relationships, because of different personalities, it takes considerably more time and effort to make the relationship work than in others. The question is, How much work do you want to invest in developing a positive relationship with your family?

A 1990 Harris poll found that 97 percent of Americans said that a happy family was their top priority, while only 60 percent said a good income was. Why then is so much more time invested in earning money than in earning and maintaining the love and respect of family members?

Behold, how good and how pleasant it is for brethren to dwell together in unity! —Psalm 133:1, NKJV

Finding the Solution to Sibling Resentment

Older kids who resent their younger siblings can make life miserable for the whole family.

Here's what often happens: the younger generally looks up to the older, while the older cruelly teases the younger or pinches him in a devious, secretive manner so the little one looks like the bad guy.

The key to a solution is to figure out why this is happening.

Could it be jealousy because the older one thinks the younger gets more parental love, attention, and gifts?

Could it be the kids spend too much time together, with not enough outside diversion?

Could it be that there is a hidden power play going on? Different personalities can aggravate this. For example, if the younger is a strong acting-out type of personality, and the older is more passive, the older may attempt to gain control of the younger through devious methods.

Could it be that the older feels he is forced to have to play with and accept his younger brother? Force never works. Not until the older can get out some of the negative feelings by talking about them will there be room for more positive feelings.

There is a way that seems right to a man, but its end is the way of death. —Proverbs 16:25, NKJV

DR. KAY KUZMA

Common Sense Parenting Makes Sense

With all the books and expert opinions available today, parents sometimes forget that they have what it takes to handle most problems: good common sense—or what I sometimes call Holy Spirit insight.

To put your common sense to work, consider what feels right to you. Think about what would be just, firm, decisive treatment that would give your children the boundaries they need to feel secure. Ask three questions to help clarify what you should do.

1. "What would I do if this were somebody else's child?" You'll find your objectivity will tend to increase as you distance yourself emotionally from your child's behavior. Then ask the second question.
2. "Why is my child acting this way?" If you can figure this out, it's a lot easier to find solutions.
3. "Am I in control of myself?"

Common sense works only when you're cool, calm, collected, and connected to Holy Spirit insight.

Get wisdom! Get understanding! —Proverbs 4:5, NKJV

Begin Eternity Today

Do you long for heaven? I do! But harps and golden crowns don't interest me nearly as much as having *time* to enjoy the beauty of the universe, *time* to spend with my family and friends, and *time* to just lie in a hammock, close my eyes, and smell the lilacs or the pine. Ah, that's eternity!

But wait a minute! Time is something God gives to us each day: twenty-four hours of it. We don't have to wait until tomorrow to enjoy eternity. Let it begin today. You can tuck a little heaven into your heart by doing something you really want to do.

Don't be like the crowd, merely existing to become "another day older and deeper in debt." There's a little piece of eternity in each day, if we'll only look for it. A friendly smile, a caring word, a whisper of fog, a shimmer of sun; it's all here on earth for us to enjoy today—if we'll take the time.

What does the worker gain from his toil? I have seen the burden God has laid on men. He has made everything beautiful in its time. He has also set eternity in the hearts of men. —Ecclesiastes 3:9–11, NIV

DR. KAY KUZMA

Counter Gangs by Meeting Needs

Gangs have a strong appeal to young people because gangs appear to give them what they value: identity, power, control, respect, excitement, belonging, and mission. When you are a member of a gang, you are *somebody*.

The problem is that these things are gained through violent, illegal, and antisocial acts. And the chance of death or imprisonment is great. Parents see the danger. Kids see only the challenge and feel the adrenaline rush they get when taking risks.

The best protection against gangs is a good home and school environment in which your kids feel they are special and incredibly important. Plan challenging—even risky—activities for them to get involved in where they can stretch their knowledge, skills, and talents to serve others rather than destroy them. Teach them how to get their needs met by living responsible lives.

Kids must experience the biblical truth, "When you give, you get," rather than the gang motto, "When you take, you get."

"It is more blessed to give than to receive." —Acts 20:35, NKJV

Children Need a Dream and a Mission

How can children gain self-respect? Doing well academically, having a good job, or being involved in sports and musical activities may help, but they're not everything.

Here's another suggestion: instead of just focusing on self, kids can gain incredible feelings of self-respect when they focus on helping others who are less fortunate through tutoring or volunteering at a community center or soup kitchen.

Your children need a dream—a mission, something to reach toward and risk their lives for. They can change the world for good if family and friends will cheer them on. Plant the spirit of optimism in your children with axioms such as, "Inch by inch, everything's a cinch." Or, "Failure is the stepping-stone to success."

Don't say, "It's impossible to make a significant difference in the lives of others because you're too young or you don't have money." Age and money are not the secrets of success; self-respect is—and it is best developed when kids focus on others rather than on self.

Where there is no vision, the people perish: but he that keepeth the law, happy is he. —Proverbs 29:18, KJV

DR. KAY KUZMA

IQ Doesn't Ensure School Success

For a child, academic success, IQ, or the class the child is in, is not as important as how he feels about himself. If a child has to struggle for grades, he'll feel dumb, even if he has a high IQ. That's one of the major reasons so many parents homeschool, at least for the first few years. They want to make sure their kids have the foundation necessary to feel competent.

Once a child gets it in his head that he isn't as smart as others, it's pretty tough to change his opinion. That's why a child needs to be placed in a school program where he has the greatest chance of success.

Children who can sit still, follow directions, do their work neatly, and pay attention have an advantage when they start school—and none of these skills has much to do with intelligence.

The key to a child's success is catching the attitude, during the first few days of school, that "I'm smart and can do it." Once a child has internalized that attitude, there's no such thing as failure.

"With God all things are possible." —Matthew 19:26, NKJV

Stop Teasing That Frightens Children

Older children love to scare younger ones by threatening them with fantasy creatures such as monsters or aliens that are going to get them. The more response the older kids get, the more it eggs them on to tease again. You've got to stop the cycle.

To the preschooler, reality and fantasy are very similar. If it looks real, it is! And because small children aren't mature enough to act brave and say, "That's pretend," and walk away without an emotional reaction, you've got to focus on changing the teasing behavior of your older ones.

Make sure there is a consequence if the older ones scare the younger. For example, confiscate any object, picture, or mask that is used to scare younger kids. Warn them that if you have to take it away, it won't be given back. Period! Don't be soft. Teasing must be stopped.

I sought the LORD, and He heard me, and delivered me from all my fears. —Psalm 34:4, NKJV

DR. KAY KUZMA

How to Avoid Bad Things

Just say No to harmful things such as drugs, alcohol, smoking, and sex before marriage. That's great advice for kids. But unfortunately, those aren't the only harmful substances that affect our children's lives. What should they do when they are confronted with something that you forgot to mention?

Here are three "commandments" that can help kids make educated decisions:

1. Don't do anything to destroy your health. Things such as eating too much fat, drinking caffeinated beverages, experimenting with marijuana, or staying up all night to study for a test fall into this category.
2. Don't do anything that will compromise your moral values, such as gambling, watching videos filled with sex and violence, or cheating on exams.
3. Don't do anything that will destroy your freedom of choice. Alcohol, smoking, and pornography are all addictive. Avoid them!

Be doers of the word, and not hearers only, deceiving yourselves. —James 1:22, NKJV

Getting Hubby's Child-Rearing Support

It's tough when you don't feel you have the child-rearing support you would like to have from your husband. Perhaps your expectations of what makes a good dad differ from his. Many men have grown up in families where Mom took care of the children while Dad worked to make sure his wife and kids were properly provided for.

Maybe your man doesn't feel very effective when it comes to the children and therefore chooses to put his energy into his job, where people look up to him and appreciate his expertise.

If your husband's ego is wrapped up in his career, you will get more cooperation from him, and he will choose to spend more time with the family, if you and the children find ways to support him and make his work easier, rather than complaining. Praise him for what he does, rather than nag about what he doesn't do. Make home a fun place to be. Men spend more time with the family when they find it rewarding.

You wives must submit to your husbands' leadership in the same way you submit to the Lord. —Ephesians 5:22, TLB

DR. KAY KUZMA

Putting People Down Won't Lift Self Up!

Sometimes conflict between Mom and Dad results from the misconception that if one parent puts the other parent down, it will make themselves look better and their children will then be closer to them. But unfortunately, this often backfires. The children not only think less of their parents when one shows disrespect for the other, but they may even take the side of the maligned.

Some parents say negative things about the other in order to justify a divorce. "If your father had been trustworthy, I wouldn't have had to leave him." In maligning the other parent, they hope their children will be able to accept the reality of the separation and not wish for reconciliation. But most children, even into adulthood, secretly still wish their parents could get back together, regardless of what may have caused the breakup.

It's interesting, but seldom does putting others down achieve the desired result. How much better it is to build up the other. How much better to remember the admonition in Philippians 4:8 (TLB): "Fix your thoughts on what is true and good and right . . . and dwell on the fine, good things in others."

Finally, brethren, whatever things are true, whatever things are noble, whatever things are just, whatever things are pure, whatever things are lovely, whatever things are of good report, if there is any virtue and if there is anything praiseworthy—meditate on these things. —Philippians 4:8, NKJV

Painting a Correct Picture of God

How can you paint a correct picture of God for your children?

Start by living a Christlike life. When you lose control or become impatient, point out that God is not like you; God is always loving and kind.

Second, let your children know that God is your best Friend; that you talk to Him, and you love sharing Jesus with others.

Then carefully select the Bible stories you tell your children, especially when they are young. In some of the Old Testament stories, it is sometimes difficult for kids to understand God's actions, so introduce them to Jesus first. After all, He came to show us what God is really like.

Finally, never threaten your children by saying that God won't love them if they disobey, or by telling them an angel writes down all the bad things they do.

You are your children's most clear picture of God, so make sure your reflection is a good one!

"I and My Father are one." —John 10:30, NKJV

DR. KAY KUZMA

"White Lie" Cheating

If your children think it's OK to cheat "just a little" to get good grades, you might use an object lesson to illustrate the effect of dishonesty.

Have them twist a paper napkin into a tight rope. Then pull it from both ends and you'll be surprised to see how strong it is. Next put a couple drops of water (representing dishonesty) in the middle and pull again. The napkin rope will break easily. This shows the effect of one dishonest act upon a person's character.

You can also help children resist the temptation to cheat by not pressuring them into always being the best. You can push children toward cheating if you have an unrealistic expectation of how well they should do.

Talk to your children about cheating, and encourage them to take a personal stand to be honest and trustworthy. Stress the fact that integrity is much more important than having the highest grades or being the best.

Fools mock at sin, but among the upright there is favor. —Proverbs 14:9, NKJV

Home Alone

Have you ever struggled with the decision of whether or not you should leave a child home alone? Age by itself is not what determines if it's safe.

There are some ten-year-olds who can be trusted home alone during the day for an hour or so, especially if it is daylight and they have something special to do, like read a good book or practice the piano. And there are some sixteen- or seventeen-year-olds who shouldn't be trusted home alone for thirty minutes!

One mom told me that when her kids were preschoolers, she had wonderful care for her children so she worked outside the home. But now that they were teenagers, she quit work. She felt the teen years were critical for moral development and the dangers of negative peer influence were the greatest. Therefore, she didn't trust anyone but herself to give her kids proper supervision.

What about leaving your children home alone? Here's safe advice: when in doubt, don't!

Whoever trusts in the LORD shall be safe. —Proverbs 29:25, NKJV

DR. KAY KUZMA

Babies Are Beautiful

Babies are beautiful, aren't they? Do you remember your first experience gazing at your newborn? You noticed that puckered mouth, the soft skin, and those perfect little fingers and toes.

Ummm. And they smelled so good—at least most of the time.

What a masterpiece of God's handiwork. What awesome potential is wrapped up in each little bundle of joy! But whether or not that potential is realized pretty much depends on you.

That's a wonderful yet frightening thought, isn't it?

But there is help available. Don't try to raise that precious child by guesswork and instinct.

Take advantage of those who have traveled this road before. Read what they write, listen to what they say, and you'll significantly increase the probability that your beautiful baby will develop into an equally beautiful person.

I will praise You, for I am fearfully and wonderfully made. —Psalm 139:14, NKJV

Rejection Can Destroy

There are two things that school-age children fear most. The first is rejection, and the second is failure. If you or your child has never suffered from feelings of peer rejection, you have no idea how devastating this can be. Love and acceptance at home helps, but it can't completely compensate for the acute pain a child feels when rejected at school.

For most children, rejection is far more painful than academic failure. A child might fail, but if she has friends who still think she's wonderful, it gives her courage to pick herself up and try again. But the value of academic success is considerably less if there are no friends with which to celebrate.

Making friends comes naturally to most, but for those children who are struggling, coach them, help them overcome abrasive habits that turn others away, encourage them to practice their social skills on one friend at a time, and point out to them the proverb, "A man [or a kid] who has friends must himself be friendly."

A man who has friends must himself be friendly, but there is a friend who sticks closer than a brother. —Proverbs 18:24, NKJV

DR. KAY KUZMA

When Kids Fear Disasters

Children get scared when they perceive a possible danger and they know they're not capable of coping with it. That's why a natural disaster can cause children overwhelming anxiety.

Children's fears are intensified by adult reactions. Any experience that is accompanied by intense emotion will tend to have a stronger and more lasting effect on a child. So watch your own reactions. Turn off the TV newscasts that keep playing the same disaster footage again and again. Focus on how people are helping others rather than on the terror of the disaster itself.

Encourage your children to talk about their fears. Here are some questions to ask them: "It's scary to think about something like this happening to you, isn't it? What is the scariest thing about it? Have you ever wondered what children your age do when they are caught in a disaster?"

It's important that you accept children's fears as real to them, even though you know they are unrealistic. Sometimes talking to others who have lived through the experience gives them ideas about how they could cope so they don't have to fear the unknown.

Yea, though I walk through the valley of the shadow of death, I will fear no evil; for You are with me; Your rod and Your staff, they comfort me. —Psalm 23:4, NKJV

Get More Out of Life With Lists

Every mother is a working mother! If you have three children, by the time your kids are eighteen years of age you will have put in eighteen thousand hours of child-generated housework. That doesn't even count the work generated by your husband! Nor does it count the time you spend chauffeuring or tucking your kids into bed! There is no such thing as a nonworking mother!

That's why mothers need lists. They can save you time and money. Get organized with a weekly list of things to do and add to it each morning.

Keep a list of easy recipes that can be made from ingredients you keep on hand.

Every time you take the last can or box of an item off the shelf, write it down on a shopping list.

List birthdays and special occasions on a calendar.

List tasks that can be done by the children.

And keep a "why-not" list of memory-making ideas and plan to do at least one a week.

Lists can definitely help you get more out of your busy life!

She watches over the ways of her household, and does not eat the bread of idleness. —Proverbs 31:27, NKJV

DR. KAY KUZMA

Humor That Hurts

The joke may be funny to you, but it could be like a knife in your child's back. Some humor hurts! Don't joke about personal things, such as your children's freckles, acne, or hairstyles. Emphasize the positive. Don't highlight things your children would rather have hidden.

And don't joke about mistakes your children have made. Mistakes are embarrassing enough. Don't add insult to injury by joking about them. Laugh with your kids, not at them.

Don't tell jokes about your children's friends. And don't tease. Younger children will believe what you say and completely miss the humor. And older ones seldom appreciate it, especially when you keep bringing it up!

So to be safe, keep your jokes on neutral things, such as sports, TV, pets, or politics, so your whole family can safely laugh together.

"Woe to you who laugh now, for you shall mourn and weep." —Luke 6:25, NKJV

Rules Are to Be Obeyed

One of the most important lessons children must learn in life if they are to grow up to be mature, law-abiding citizens, is that if they disobey the rules there are consequences. That's why it's important that parents support a school system that is trying to teach this lesson.

Sometimes the school rules may seem ridiculous. And sometimes they may be difficult to keep because of a child's personality characteristics and previous behavior. But a rule is a rule, and the person in charge has the responsibility to enforce it.

If your kids don't like a rule, instead of disobeying, encourage them to get involved in school government and see if it can be changed through the democratic process.

If your children have to suffer a consequence, let them know that learning the lesson that there are consequences for disobedience is probably the most important lesson they will ever have to learn. So encourage them to grin and bear it—and learn it as quickly as possible!

I delight to do Your will, O my God, and Your law is within my heart. —Psalm 40:8, NKJV

DR. KAY KUZMA

Invitation Etiquette

I received a letter from a grandmother who gave some wise counsel. She wrote, "Invitations passed out at school to a select group of children nearly destroyed me when I was a child. I cried for two days because I wasn't invited to a birthday party. My daughter lived through this same experience a time or two, and I watched her suffer. Now it's happened to my grandson. Invitations were passed out in school to a select group of children. When he asked where his invitation was, the comment was made, 'You don't get any. I don't like you.'"

She ends her letter with this request, "Please tell parents that if children want to celebrate their birthdays with their classmates, let them bring cupcakes to school for everyone. But if they want to have a birthday party with a select group of friends, send the invitations to the children's homes and encourage them to not talk about the upcoming party at school. It's too hard on the children who aren't invited."

"Show mercy and compassion everyone to his brother." —Zechariah 7:9, NKJV

Show Appreciation

I once analyzed a number of research studies on the traits of strong, healthy families and found that showing appreciation ranked next to the top. Showing appreciation is good for others, but it is also good for your own emotional health. As you look for the good in others and express what you appreciate, your mind is bathed in positive, healing emotions.

Regardless of what you may think, you can find something good in everyone, including obnoxious family members. Notice the person's appearance and mention something you do like. Smile or wave to acknowledge the person's existence. Let them see in your body language and words that they are special. Compliment their skills and abilities. When a difficult moral choice is made, let them know you admire their integrity. We all crave this kind of recognition.

It doesn't cost anything to show appreciation, so give it generously.

You open Your hand and satisfy the desire of every living thing. —Psalm 145:16, NKJV

DR. KAY KUZMA

Betrayed by Friends

Few things in this world can cause children more emotional pain than when a family member or friend betrays them and spreads lies about them. If you discover your child is a victim of this cruelty, encourage your child to not stoop to their level. Tell them the following: "Don't malign others for maligning you. Truth has a way of surfacing in time, if you hold your head high.

"Watch your words and actions carefully so you can avoid all appearances of 'inappropriate' behavior. Don't give anyone more ammunition to hurt you.

"And don't retreat. Keep attending group functions, even if you think others may be talking about you. If you withdraw and aren't there to defend yourself, they will likely talk behind your back.

"If someone confronts you, kindly offer them the truth, but don't get defensive. Defensiveness is often perceived as an admission of guilt.

"And pray for them who 'say all manner of evil against you falsely.' "

"Blessed are you when they revile you and persecute you, and say all kinds of evil against you falsely for My sake." —Matthew 5:11, NKJV

Give Permission to Debate

For some kids, debate comes naturally. Parents say one thing and kids counter with another opinion. The problem for parents is to know when children have a legitimate complaint and can offer a reasonable solution to a problem if they are given an audience, and when they are just trying to control the situation.

It never hurts to give children permission to present their case. But parents need to be in control. Arguing for the sake of arguing can become a dysfunctional habit. So as soon as kids start to argue with you, say, "I can tell you have a strong opinion about this. You need to understand Mom and Dad make the decisions in this area, but we are willing to hear what you have to say. But after we listen, discuss the issue, and finally make a decision, that's it! No more arguing!"

Healthy families allow their children to freely discuss differences in opinion, but they don't allow their kids to control them by arguing so much that they wear down their patience and they finally give in.

My son, hear the instruction of your father, and do not forsake the law of your mother.
—Proverbs 1:8, NKJV

DR. KAY KUZMA

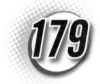

Don't Interrupt to Correct

It's interesting how many rules we require our children to obey that we ourselves break! For example, the rule, "Don't interrupt."

Your child comes home excited about the game. "Dad, you'll never believe what happened, this here guy at school, a real sharp—"

"Don't say, 'this here.' Say 'this guy.' "

"OK, OK. Just listen, Dad. This here—I mean this guy at school who is a real sharp dude, just got a—"

"Dude? What kind of a name is that?"

"Dad, just listen. This guy, who's sharp as hell, just got a contract for—"

"And don't swear!"

"Never mind, Dad. It's not that important anyway."

Let me ask you, what good is perfect English if, in your push to perfection, you squelch your child's speech so often that he clams up and never uses it when you're around?

Let your speech always be with grace, seasoned with salt, that you may know how you ought to answer each one.
—Colossians 4:6, NKJV

The VIP Method of Building Character

When I say "VIP," you automatically think of a very important person, but the initials *VIP* can also stand for three of the most important things parents need to provide for their children's character development.

Wholesome character traits don't happen by chance. It takes Vision, Inspiration, and a good Positive Pattern. That's V for Vision, I for Inspiration, and P for Positive Pattern. Here's how it works:

You must give your children a vision of what they can become. Children tend to live up to their parents' expectations.

Children also need inspiration or motivation to choose right from wrong and to develop their potential.

And finally, every child needs a positive pattern or role model.

With Vision, Inspiration, and a Positive Pattern, your child can become a VIP.

Imitate me, just as I also imitate Christ. —1 Corinthians 11:1, NKJV

DR. KAY KUZMA

INDEX

INDEX

INDEX

INDEX